# Alcohol Tolerance
# and Social Drinking

# THE GUILFORD SUBSTANCE ABUSE SERIES

### Editors

## HOWARD T. BLANE, Ph.D.
*Research Institute on Alcoholism, Buffalo*

## THOMAS R. KOSTEN, M.D.
*Yale University School of Medicine, New Haven*

# ALCOHOL TOLERANCE AND SOCIAL DRINKING
## Learning the Consequences

MURIEL VOGEL-SPROTT
*University of Waterloo*

**THE GUILFORD PRESS**
**New York    London**

© 1992 The Guilford Press
A Division of Guilford Publications, Inc.
72 Spring Street, New York, NY 10012

Printed in the United States of America

This book is printed on acid-free paper.

Last digit is print number: 9 8 7 6 5 4 3 2 1

Library of Congress Cataloging-in-Publication Data
Vogel-Sprott, Muriel.
    Alcohol tolerance and social drinking: learning the consequences
  / Muriel Vogel-Sprott.
        p.    cm. – (The Guilford substance abuse series)
    Includes bibliographical reference and index.
    ISBN 0-89862-191-7
    1. Alcohol–Physiological effect.   2. Drinking of alcoholic
  beverages.   3. Drug tolerance.   4. Alcoholism.   5. Expectation
  (Psychology)  I. Title.  II. Series.
    [DNLM: 1. Alcohol Drinking–psychology.   2. Alcohol, Ethyl.
  3. Drug Tolerance–physiology.     QV 38 V879a]
  QP801.A3V64   1992
  615'.7828–dc20
  DNLM/DLC
  for Library of Congress                                    91-35422
                                                                  CIP

*To David, always*

# *Preface*

Newspaper headlines and public
heath reports continually remind us that many individuals in society
abuse alcohol. One characteristic that correlates with alcohol abuse is
a high degree of tolerance for the drug. Thus it is often thought that
tolerance may increase the risk of alcohol abuse because alcohol
consumption would have to increase to reinstate the effects initially
attained by lower doses.

It is clear that an understanding of the mechanisms of tolerance
will require research on the pharmacological action of alcohol and the
pathological physiological, neurochemical, or other biological states
ensuing from excessive exposure to alcohol. An equally clear question, but less researched, is why most drinkers can use alcohol
without making the transition from social to abusive drinking. To the
extent that tolerance contributes to the risk of alcohol abuse, an
understanding of the factors inducing tolerance in nonproblem
drinkers becomes crucial. This book was prompted by the need to
know about the alcohol tolerance of ordinary social drinkers.

The Introduction and Background sections of the book explain
the reasons for an interest in the alcohol tolerance of social drinkers.
These sections contain basic information about alcohol and theories of
tolerance, and present a historical perspective on the seemingly
anomalous and neglected view that tolerance is affected by events
*after* drinking. The third section presents an analysis of this possibility
and provides the theoretical framework for the experiments described
in the next two sections. The studies demonstrate that the expected
consequence of behavior under alcohol influences social drinkers'

acquisition of tolerance, its transfer to new tasks, and its extinction in spite of continuing drinking occasions. The research also shows that these learned expectancies are portable in that mental rehearsal of the consequence of behavior under alcohol affects tolerance the same way as does firsthand performance and experience of the consequence. An extension of the investigation indicates that these expected consequences have a similar effect on resistance to the impairing effect of a single dose of alcohol. In sum, the evidence suggests that the behavioral tolerance of social drinkers resembles adaptive learning and may be a very common, normal phenomenon. The final sections discuss the implications of the findings for new research, and for social problems. Impaired driving, the role that tolerance may play in encouraging alcohol abuse, and the ramifications for treatment and prevention are discussed. An overview relates our conclusions to contemporary views and issues of alcohol use and misuse.

Most research has examined tolerance as a potential indicator of pathology. This book is unique in presenting a systematic investigation of tolerance in normal states represented by nonproblem social drinking. Thus the information presented in this book could be of broad interest to scientists from many different disciplines as well as graduate or senior undergraduates who may wish to conduct research on alcohol's effects on humans. Therefore, I have tried to avoid the technical terminology of psychology as much as possible. When such terms are used, I have taken care to explain them as simply and clearly as possible. The abbreviated nature of published articles does not permit a full explanation of experimental procedures, and drug experiments with humans require special, subtle skills that are not as well known or obvious as those in animal or biological research. Therefore, I have included detailed information on the methodology in a chapter that could serve as an instruction manual to aid others who would like to perform alcohol experiments with humans.

More generally, the book is intended to present information that scientifically minded readers can appreciate, and weigh for themselves. It is this evaluation process that best guarantees the evolution of better research contributions to knowledge.

It has been my good fortune to have a number of graduate students who have been interested in the puzzle of behavioral tolerance to alcohol in humans. Most of the research described in the book is a result of our collaboration. Although writing a book is a solitary pursuit, it involves the support and help of many others. Much of the book was prepared in Guanajuato, Mexico, where Dr. J. A. Canavati, Director of the Centro de Investigaciones en Matemáticas, generously offered the resources of the institution, and Laura Rincón Gallardo provided much help. I have greatly appreciated the advice and encouragement of Dr. H. Blane, Director of the Research Institute on Alcoholism, Buffalo, New York. I am especially grateful for reviews and helpful comments on drafts of the book by Professors G. E. MacKinnon and D. A. Sprott of the University of Waterloo, and Dr. R. E. Mann of the Addiction Research Foundation. Thanks are due to Jane Sprott for the masterful preparation of the figures in the book. I am also indebted to many students who so ably played the role of critic. These people include Tina Adam, Paul Fera, Mark Fillmore, Eleanor Liu, Michael Staines, Martin Zack, and Marna Zinatelli.

MURIEL VOGEL-SPROTT

# Contents

# *Alcohol Tolerance and Social Drinking*

# 1

# INTRODUCTION

For decades researchers have investigated the problem of alcohol abuse and alcoholism. As this work has continued, and solutions remain elusive, some workers have begun to wonder if the research problem has been too narrowly defined. It is not just that we have trouble understanding and controlling the evolution of alcohol abuse and alcoholism, we do not know much about social drinking either. Factors that may stabilize social drinking or foster its transition to abusive drinking have not been construed as part of the research endeavor in the past. The last decade has seen more frequent expression of the view that understanding factors associated with "normal" social drinking may provide new information that could greatly aid efforts to prevent and treat alcohol abuse. In a sense, this notion is akin to the old adage, "You can't fix something unless you know how it worked in the first place."

A thorough investigation of the many facets of social drinking will require research by many disciplines. But work is starting, and some exciting pieces of the puzzle are beginning to be identified. This book describes the pursuit of one thread of the mystery, the development of behavioral tolerance to alcohol. The research is designed to test factors that may cause social drinkers to display tolerance.

Tolerance was singled out for investigation because it is a ubiquitous phenomenon. The term is familiar to most people. *Webster's New Collegiate Dictionary* (1973) defines tolerance as "the capacity to endure or resist the action of a drug." However, experiments use a precise operational definition that will be presented in the next

1

chapter. Tolerance is an important consideration in medical practice because the initial beneficial effect of a drug treatment sometimes diminishes when the drug is repeatedly administered. In these cases the dose may have to be increased to maintain the desired effect. Unfortunately, larger doses of a drug are also more likely to evoke other unwanted effects. Thus, from a medical perspective, drug tolerance is altogether undesirable and poses impediments to the efficacy of any prolonged drug treatment regimen.

Drug tolerance is also observed when drugs are used for nonmedical or recreational purposes. Ethanol—"alcohol"—is a prime example. Habitual users of alcohol commonly display minimal effects of a dose that would evoke an intense reaction in a naive user. The occurrence of alcohol tolerance is also considered undesirable because higher doses of alcohol may be required to maintain the effects initially achieved with smaller doses. Thus the development of alcohol tolerance is suspected to encourage an escalation of drinking, and to pose a risk of alcohol abuse. Higher doses result in prolonged higher concentrations of alcohol in the body. This increased exposure to alcohol is thought to be accompanied by physiological changes that culminate in physical dependence, so that withdrawal symptoms occur when the drug is withheld.

Tolerance is usually assumed to develop gradually over years of continued drug use. However, the degree to which such drug exposure can completely account for the tolerance of humans cannot be tested experimentally because ethical considerations preclude such long-term administration of alcohol. Indirect evidence, such as the high degree of behavioral tolerance to alcohol that characterizes alcoholics, is consistent with the drug exposure notion. However, the adequacy of this information is limited by the fact that alcoholics are distinguished from the general population of drinkers only *after* the disorder is diagnosed. All of the important information concerning the prior growth of their tolerance is missing. Thus the role that alcohol tolerance may play in moving an individual from a social to an abusive drinker is unknown. Answers to this question require an understanding of factors that affect the alcohol tolerance of individuals who are beginning their social drinking career and are not yet identified as alcohol abusers or alcoholics.

Personal experience and observations of others suggest that tolerance to the behavioral effects of alcohol can occur during early stages in its social use. Factors causing the development of this early form of tolerance may be particularly important in understanding the course of social drinking. In this book, findings on behavioral tolerance that have appeared in the literature are integrated with the results of a research program conducted with colleagues at the University of Waterloo. The evidence and its implications offer a different perspective for understanding factors affecting the alcohol tolerance of social drinkers and new insights on the role their tolerance may play in promoting drug abuse.

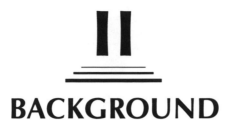

# BACKGROUND

# 1

## Ethanol:
## The Beverage Alcohol

Chemistry distinguishes several types of alcohols. Some members of the alcohol family are methyl alcohol (methanol), isopropyl alcohol, and ethyl alcohol (ethanol). The first two alcohols are toxic and would only be consumed accidentally. Ethanol is the substance people drink, under the familiar name of alcohol. The term *alcohol* is used in this book to refer to ethanol. Beverages containing alcohol have been used since the dawn of history and have played a persistent role in the activities of humankind. Ancient civilizations used alcohol to facilitate religious and social activities, enhance pleasure, and reduce pain. Contemporary society uses alcohol for similar purposes.

The widespread use of alcohol throughout the centuries is likely due not only to its attractive effects, but also to its availability. Low concentrations of alcohol, about 10% by volume, are produced in nature through fermentation by yeast of sugars that are present in many vegetables, fruits, and grains. Modern methods of fermentation use special yeasts rather than the wild variety, but the fermentation process still yields beverages with low concentrations of alcohol. Higher concentrations can be produced by distillation processes involved in the manufacture of liquor or spirits.

### Preliminary Considerations

Our review of alcohol will provide background information needed to consider the various explanations of behavioral tolerance to the drug.

7

More detailed reviews of the chemical and pharmacological properties of alcohol are available elsewhere (e.g., Ritchie, 1985). One
comprehensive assessment of the effect of alcohol on human performance and behavior has been provided by Wallgren and Barry (1971).

## Administration

Humans customarily administer alcohol orally. The alcohol is absorbed into the blood from the stomach lining and upper intestine.
Alcohol provides energy as calories, but contains no vitamins. The
sole elements of alcohol are carbon, hydrogen, and oxygen, and its
chemical formula is $C_2H_5OH$. The alcohol molecule is comparatively
small. In contrast to many psychoactive drugs, alcohol is highly water
soluble. Its oil–water partition coefficient is just high enough for it to
pass the blood–brain barrier, but low enough that it is not fat soluble.
Therefore, alcohol enters the central nervous system quite quickly
and is fairly evenly distributed throughout all body fluids and tissues,
including those of the brain (Julien, 1981).

In research with humans, blood alcohol concentration (BAC) is
usually estimated from breath samples and measured in mg alcohol
per 100 ml blood. This unit of measurement is used throughout the
book. BAC measures are sometimes also expressed in terms of
percentages. For example, a BAC of 80 mg/100 ml is equivalent to a
BAC of 0.08%. In many jurisdictions, 0.08% is the legal definition of
intoxication.

Alcohol is absorbed most rapidly when given in a 15–30%
solution by volume. The rate at which BAC rises is also greatly
affected by the contents of the stomach and the rate of drinking.
Swifter-rising BACs are obtained under fasting conditions and when
alcohol is consumed more quickly. Under such conditions, peak
BACs can occur within 30 minutes after drinking stops. As with other
drugs, the actual peak plasma concentration resulting from a dose of
alcohol depends upon a drinker's body weight and composition.

Individuals of the same weight who have proportionately more
body fat attain higher BACs because their total fluid volume for the
distribution of alcohol is less. This results in a higher concentration of
alcohol in the blood. The body composition of women is characterized
by proportionately more fat than men. As a result, women tend to
have a smaller volume of distribution than men. A given mg/kg dose
of alcohol will yield a higher peak BAC in women.

The nature of the alcoholic beverage also can affect the absorption rate. Carbonation hastens absorption, probably by forcing the
alcohol more quickly into the small intestine where a greater surface

area allows more rapid absorption. Although the degree of carbonation in a drink may seem a comparatively trivial consideration, it can create a surprising increase in the peak BAC attained. My effort to solve the mysterious case of the homemade champagne provides a good example of this point.

The making of champagne requires a meticulous mathematical precision in the measurement of sugar and yeasts, timing of fermenting, and racking. It is a hobby that is well suited to the temperament of my statistician husband. He creates an elixir whose appearance and taste equal that of commercial domestic champagne. Moreover, it has an enduring carbonation that more closely resembles true French champagne. However, I suspected that the homemade version had a higher alcoholic content than the commercial domestic beverage because it seemed to yield much stronger alcohol effects. But detailed descriptions of the exact amount of sugar and yeast added, the constraints on fermentation and hygrometer measures of alcohol content suggested that the homemade and commercial beverages must have the same alcohol content. Based on logic and diplomacy, it seemed best to abandon my subversive allegation concerning the homemade champagne. So the mystery remained until it was agreed that an experiment with myself as subject could provide the solution. I spent two evenings drinking champagne, the homemade version one night, and the commercial beverage another. In each case, drinking began after a 4-hour fast, and a dose of 0.55 g/kg was consumed within the same time limit. Such a dose would be likely to raise the BAC to a peak of around 55 to 60 mg/100 ml, and would provide a good opportunity to examine the rising and peak BACs obtained with each beverage. After drinking ceased, measures of BAC were obtained from breath samples, and the results are shown in Figure 1.

The commercial champagne yielded a peak BAC of 70 mg/100 ml, slightly higher than expected. The homemade champagne generated an astonishing high of 90 mg/100 ml. The evidence vindicated my suspicion. Fortunately, the results also reflected favorably on the authenticity of the homemade champagne. Its greater enduring carbonation was more comparable to the French version, whose potent intoxicating effects are legendary. The experiment also restored domestic harmony, but that is another story.

## Human Performance and Behavior

Alcohol is structurally related to ether and classified pharmacologically as a general depressant. It is capable of inducing a general

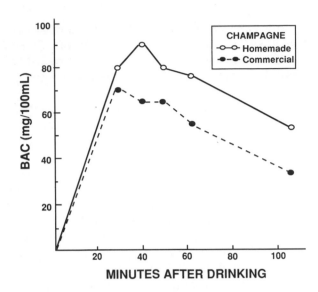

**FIGURE 1.** Blood alcohol concentrations (BACs) from two champagnes having the same alcohol content but differing in carbonation.

reversible depression of the central nervous system. The effects of alcohol on humans are familiar to most people, owing to personal experience or observations of other drinkers. There is a vast amount of research examining the detrimental effects of alcohol on human vision, vigilance, complex reaction time, eye–hand coordination, balance (body sway), gait, mental concentration, and problem solving (Wallgren & Barry, 1971). Slight deficits in some of these behaviors may be observed when BAC is as low as 20 mg/100 ml, but impairment is more likely to occur when blood levels are over 50 mg/100 ml. When BAC is between 50 to 100 mg/100 ml, social drinkers appear more talkative, cheerful, and boisterous. When the peak BAC has been attained and plasma levels begin to decline, drinkers may become tired and sleepy.

Although there is some correlation between blood alcohol levels and the drug's behavioral and emotional effects, there is also a considerable lack of correspondence. The causes of this discrepancy are not well understood. Some inconsistencies between a drinker's BAC and the observed effect may have to do with the type of effect a drinker expects alcohol to have (Hull & Bond, 1986). The influence of this and other sorts of learned expectancies is a particularly important consideration in the research described in later chapters.

Acute tolerance, sometimes termed "tachyphylaxis," is another factor that could disturb the correlation between a BAC and its effect.

*Acute tolerance* refers to the observation that the intensity of the effect of a given BAC is typically more pronounced when blood alcohol levels are rising than when they are falling (Ritchie, 1985). It resembles an adaptive reaction, and it is commonly attributed to some rapidly occurring homeostatic adjustments in neural membranes to the presence of alcohol (Grilly, 1989). Research considering the adequacy of this explanation will be discussed in Chapter 8.

There is much folklore about the effect of drinking alcohol. An amusing old fable about the monk who introduced grapes to France provides a good caricature of alcohol effects.

> At first, the vine was hidden in the bone of a bird, then, after outgrowing the bird, it was hidden in the bone of a lion and finally, in the bone of a donkey. Later after the vine had grown and wine was made, the monks who drank it showed the characteristics of the animals used in its transportation. After the first bottle they sang like birds, after the second, they had the courage of lions, but after the third they behaved like asses. (McKim, 1991, p. 96)

The effects of the third bottle of wine in the fable illustrates the toxic behavioral effects of alcohol. At this stage, a drinker's activities could have hazardous consequences, even though the BAC is still below toxic physiological levels. Gross physical and behavioral symptoms of intoxication are usually displayed when BAC reaches levels over 150 mg/100 ml. Social drinkers may be quite nauseated and begin to be lethargic and stuporous. Most persons would become unconscious at a BAC of 350 mg/100 ml, and death from alcohol poisoning is likely to occur when BAC is near 500 mg/100 ml. Lethal BACs require an extremely large intake of alcohol. For example, to attain a BAC of 500 mg/100 ml, an ordinary-sized male (75 kg; 165 lb) would have to drink 42 oz (1,193 ml) of 40% liquor. In terms of drinks containing 1.5 oz (43 ml) of liquor, this amounts to 28 drinks. Unless the alcohol is consumed very quickly, lethal BACs are unlikely to occur, because a drinker would ordinarily vomit and pass out before such a huge amount of alcohol could be consumed.

## Neuropharmacology

In contrast to many drugs that interact with a receptor site to alter the function of a synapse, no specific receptor site has been identified for alcohol. Evidence suggests that alcohol affects cell membranes and alters their fluidity, causing a swelling that in turn disturbs many properties of membranes and alters many aspects of conduction and synaptic neurotransmission (Chin & Goldstein, 1981).

The longstanding search for some drug that could act as a competitive antagonist to alcohol and block its effects has so far been fruitless (McKim, 1991). The most recent candidate for an antialcohol pill is a substance identified as Ro15-4513. This chemical is a derivative of the benzodiazepine class of drugs, of which diazepam, known by its trade name Valium, is also a member. Some work (Suzdak et al., 1986) on the neurotransmitter *γ-aminobuytric acid (GABA)* suggests that the alcohol effect on disordering membrane lipids results in enhanced activity of GABA at its receptors, and Ro15-4513 may block most of the action of alcohol at GABA receptors. If Ro15-4513 blocks the effect of alcohol at GABA receptors, it may explain the reduced behavioral symptoms of alcohol intoxication in Ro15-4513 treated animals. It is not yet clear whether these effects are produced because Ro15-4513 acts as a specific antagonist or is just another drug that has pharmacological effects opposite to alcohol (Britton, Ehlers, & Koob, 1988; Suzdak et al., 1988). The effect of Ro15-4513 on behavioral symptoms of intoxication in humans has not yet been reported. However, it is clear that Ro15-4513 is not a practical cure for the intoxicating effects of overindulgence, and it does not alter the dose of alcohol that induces lethal effects. If the drug were taken before imbibing, a drinker could consume a lethal amount of alcohol without the restraining influence of intoxication.

Recent research on receptor-gated ion channels using glutamate receptors and the glutamate receptor agonist N-methyl-D-aspartate (NMDA) suggests that alcohol also may inhibit ion currents activated by transmitter substances (Lovinger, White, & Weight, 1989). Investigations of the effect of alcohol on other receptor-gated ion channels are continuing. It seems that the ongoing research on alcohol continues to support the conclusion that the range of biological phenomena affected directly and indirectly by ethanol is extremely large (Kalant, LeBlanc, & Gibbins, 1971).

## Metabolism

The enzyme alcohol dehydrogenase (ADH) converts alcohol to acetaldehyde, and is the first step in the metabolism of alcohol. The metabolism of alcohol depends primarily upon ADH in the liver. However, research has identified ADH in the stomach that could begin to metabolize alcohol before it enters the bloodstream and is carried to the liver (DiPadova, Worner, Julkunen, & Lieber, 1987). Evidence for this "first pass" gastric metabolism by ADH has been provided by showing that the peak BAC from an oral dose of alcohol is lower than that obtained by bypassing the stomach with an intravenous injection of the same dose.

Gastric ADH is now the subject of much research, and the interpretation of the evidence is becoming controversial. Frezza et al. (1990) reported that women have a decreased gastric ADH activity compared to men. Since women also tend to have a smaller volume of distribution for alcohol, their reduced gastric ADH would further operate to cause women to have higher peak BACs than men of the same size receiving the same dose. This led Frezza et al. to suggest that the decreased gastric ADH of women may explain the increased tissue damage and medical problems among alcoholic women as compared with alcoholic men. But this speculation has been challenged by evidence that gastric ADH changes with age, *increasing* in women and *decreasing* in men. Among drinkers over the age of 50, women have higher gastric ADH than men (Seitz, Egerer, & Simanowski, 1990). In addition, York (1990) has pointed out that the alcohol consumption of women does not usually match that of men, drink per drink. He provided evidence on alcohol intake based upon body weight that suggested alcoholic women report drinking only 61–73% as much alcohol as men. Thus York suggested that women may choose to consume less alcohol because of greater bioavailability of the drug in their blood. In other words, rather than matching the per-kg dose of men, women may be drinking to match the BACs of men. Evidence suggesting that male and female social drinkers do administer alcohol to attain equivalent BACs was obtained some time ago in our laboratory (Shortt & Vogel-Sprott, 1978). In this study a group of men and women attended four "cocktail parties" to drink an unfamiliar punch on some occasions and a known alcoholic beverage on others. On each occasion the drinkers' BACs were measured when they decided they had reached their "stopping point" for drinking. When the drinkers stopped, their average BAC was 50 mg/100 ml and there was no detectable difference between the BACs of men and women.

The metabolism rate of most drugs increases when there is a higher concentration of the drug in the blood. However, alcohol differs in that the rate of metabolism is fairly linear with time, and independent of BAC. The average alcohol elimination rate of humans is estimated to be about 16 mg/100 ml per hour (Kalant, 1971; Kopun & Propping, 1977). However, rates as low as 10 and as high as 34 mg/100 ml per hour have been observed in normal healthy individuals (Coldwell & Smith, 1959; Harger & Forney, 1963). There are substantial differences in elimination rates among individuals (Li,

1983), and some of this variation may be genetically determined (Kopun & Propping, 1977).

Various dietary and environmental factors that may accelerate the elimination of alcohol have been extensively studied. Research has also investigated the effect of an additional source of metabolism, termed the *microsomal ethanol oxidizing system (MEOS)*. The MEOS metabolizes a small amount of alcohol, and this activity may increase slightly in the presence of continuously high blood alcohol levels (McKim, 1991). However, neither the MEOS nor dietary nor environmental factors have been found to have any clinically significant effect on the metabolism of alcohol (Julien, 1981). Research indicates that the metabolic rate is subject to little alteration because it has a definite and quickly attained upper limit (Jaffe, 1970, p. 292).

In summary, although alcohol is one of the oldest drugs known to humankind, it seems still to be one of the most enigmatic. It acts everywhere in general, and nowhere in particular. Once in the bloodstream, there is no agent that can be administered to block its effects, and no effective means of hastening its elimination. Instances of behavioral tolerance to alcohol are an equally fascinating puzzle.

## The Definition of Alcohol Tolerance

It is well known that regular drinkers generally are able to tolerate larger amounts of alcohol. This meaning of tolerance is conveyed in dictionary definitions. However, experimenters use a precise, operational definition of tolerance. In order to demonstrate an increase in tolerance within the same individual, some specific drug effect is initially measured. Drug exposures are then repeated. When a readministration of the same dose produces *less* of an effect, the occurrence of tolerance is inferred. This phenomenon is sometimes termed "chronic" tolerance to distinguish it from acute tolerance that is observed during declining BACs following a single dose of alcohol.

Tolerance may also be inferred by demonstrating a shift to the right in the dose response curve. That is, the effect of a larger dose produces the degree of effect initially obtained with a lower dose. This evidence is needed when tolerance is tested after extended exposure to massive doses of alcohol, because the debilitating stress and exhaustion created by an intense dosing regimen may also reduce responsiveness. Usually, these circumstances only arise in animal experiments.

There is good agreement among researchers concerning the

observations required to claim the occurrence of tolerance. However, investigators from various disciplines tend to favor different explanations of the processes involved in tolerance. Thus disagreements arise over the necessary and sufficient conditions that induce tolerance during the intervening period between the initial and final measure of drug effects. One view that may be familiar to readers is that tolerance results solely from drug use. More exposure will create more tolerance. This assumption evolved from research in the biological sciences, and is still widely accepted. However, investigations of drug tolerance by other disciplines have increased exponentially during the past decade (Goudie & Emmett-Oglesby, 1989), and evidence accumulated by this research indicates that factors other than the drug also profoundly affect tolerance. Drug exposure alone cannot provide an adequate explanation of the phenomenon. Much of this evidence has been obtained from research with alcohol, and here even more extreme objections to a drug-induced biological explanation of tolerance have been advanced. Some behavioral scientists (Wenger, Tiffany, Bombardier, Nicholls, & Woods, 1981) have argued that the development of alcohol tolerance is triggered by learning about the drug effect, and that drug exposure is only incidental.

Current research suggests that the development of alcohol tolerance is much more complex than first believed. Oddly enough, as more factors are found to affect tolerance, it becomes more difficult to determine the specific events needed to produce it.

## Biological Explanations of Alcohol Tolerance

Because research in the behavioral sciences evolved more slowly than in chemistry and pharmacology, theories of drug tolerance based upon the findings of the biological disciplines were developed early and have become widely accepted. These "traditional" views provide a background upon which to understand the emergence of contemporary views of alcohol tolerance.

Pharmacology has identified two important biological processes that could operate to enhance tolerance to some drugs. These two processes are known as *dispositional* or *pharmacokinetic tolerance*, and *functional* or *pharmacodynamic tolerance*. Extensive research has investigated the role of each in the occurrence of alcohol tolerance.

### Dispositional Tolerance

A reduction in the effect of a drug owing to an increased rate of elimination is termed dispositional tolerance. The drug effect is weaker because the clearance of alcohol is hastened and the duration of drug action is therefore abbreviated. Pharmacokinetic tolerance to alcohol has been indicated by some research with animals and humans that found chronic ingestion of high doses of alcohol may slightly increase the capacity to metabolize the drug (Hawkins, Kalant, & Khanna, 1966; Isbell, Fraser, Wikler, Belleville, & Eisenmann, 1955; Mendelson, Stein, & Mello, 1965). However, this effect on metabolism is not very robust because the elimination rates of alcoholics are within the range obtained from normal healthy individuals. A valuable assessment of the possible occurrence of pharmacokinetic tolerance to alcohol has been provided in experiments by Truitt (1971). He measured blood acetaldehyde and metabolism for 5 hours after administering a moderate dose of alcohol to age-matched alcoholics and nonalcoholics. All subjects were healthy volunteers. The alcoholics were patients in an alcoholism clinic. In assessing his findings, and that of others, Truitt concluded, "Several indications for faster metabolism [in alcoholics] can be found, but these are obscured by the wide variation in both alcoholic and nonalcoholic drinkers" (1971, p. 223).

In general, the work on alcohol metabolism has suggested that dispositional tolerance is unlikely to contribute to an understanding of the development of alcohol tolerance. At best, dispositional tolerance could only operate to abbreviate the action of alcohol, and this could not account for the degree of tolerance that alcoholics display during both absorption and elimination phases of a dose. Moreover, it cannot explain why chronic alcoholics occasionally manifest severe symptoms of intoxication under comparatively small doses of alcohol to which they had previously displayed tolerance. This "reverse tolerance" was described by Jellinek (1960), who speculated that it was due to a nutritionally debilitating lifestyle and general weakened state of ill health. Although explanations of reverse tolerance remain speculative, research consistent with Jellinek's opinion has shown that chronic alcohol consumption in rats accelerated gastric emptying, which in turn decreased gastric ADH activity (Gentry, Baraona, & Lieber, 1990). A reduction in gastric ADH would reduce the amount of alcohol metabolized in the stomach, so that more alcohol would be available to enter the blood. Under these circumstances, a given dose of alcohol would yield higher BACs. These findings suggest that the reverse tolerance occasionally displayed by some alcoholics may, in part, reflect an impairment of metabolism that increases the bioavailability of alcohol and results in higher BACs and more intense symptoms.

The studies on dispositional tolerance to alcohol have led to the conclusion that this process is quite unlikely to explain why individuals habituated to alcohol are little affected at a BAC that produces severe effects in drug-naive users. The conclusion in turn has encouraged the assumption that alcohol tolerance must result from some type of drug-induced reaction that is opposite in direction to the drug effect and thus serves to compensate by restoring homeostasis (Kalant, 1987). The compensatory response is most usually attributed to some form of adaptation to the drug's action by the nervous system, and this form of tolerance is commonly called *functional tolerance* (Kalant, 1987).

## Functional Tolerance

This view of tolerance attributes the phenomenon to a physiological homeostatic reaction to the direct pharmacological action of the drug (e.g., Collier, 1965). The same compensatory adaptive process has also been assumed to underlie *physical dependence*. Physical dependence in a habitual drug user is identified by withholding the drug and observing the occurrence of distressing *withdrawal symptoms* that are primarily opposite in nature to the drug effect. Because alcohol sedates and depresses many functions, alcohol withdrawal is characterized by symptoms of hyperexcitability, such as tremors or seizures.

The notion that a common compensatory reaction causes tolerance and physical dependence is parsimonious and has considerable intuitive appeal. The reasoning is as follows: When the drug is present, the compensatory adaptive response restores normal function so tolerance is observed. Withholding the drug unmasks the compensatory reaction that is manifested as withdrawal symptoms. From this perspective, tolerance and physical dependence are a consequence of drug exposure and are manifestations of a physiological adaptive process that is specific to the type of drug and its mechanism of action (Kalant, 1987). Research on opiates has provided considerable support for these assumptions, and the viewpoint has become prevalent and extrapolated to alcohol. "There can now be little doubt that ethanol tolerance and physical dependence are closely related phenomena which develop essentially in parallel in man" (Kalant, 1975, p. 5). The wide acceptance of the notion that tolerance and physical dependence represent an equivalent process is also evident in the American Psychiatric Association's (1987) definition of alcoholism, where symptoms of physical dependence *or* tolerance to alcohol on the part of a patient can contribute equally to the diagnosis of alcoholism.

The notion of a physiological adaptive reaction triggered by exposure of the central nervous system to the action of alcohol offers a neat, parsimonious explanation for tolerance and dependence. But this explanation encounters problems. The attribution of tolerance and physical dependence to the same process implies that they should be correlated within the same individual. Yet it is not uncommon for habitual heavy users of alcohol to display great tolerance with no symptoms of physical dependence (Jellinek, 1960). The assumption that tolerance reflects an adaptation to alcohol by the nervous system suggests tolerance should occur fairly equally to all effects of the drug. Yet this is seldom observed. It is acknowledged that an individual may display a high degree of tolerance to some effects of alcohol, and no tolerance to other effects (Kalant et al., 1971). Research with alcohol-habituated and alcohol-naive animals leads to the same conclusion. Alcohol-habituated animals can display more tolerance to some effects of alcohol when their tolerance to a lethal dose of alcohol does not differ appreciably from that of alcohol-naive animals (Jaffe, 1970, p. 280).

The uneven development of tolerance to specific effects of alcohol has led to the proposal that the alcohol-induced compensatory reaction underlying tolerance is specific to the functional disturbance created (Kalant, 1987). This proposal may help to explain why tolerance occurs to some effects of alcohol and not others. However, major difficulties with the assumption entailed in functional tolerance remain. There is no evidence as yet that alcohol causes an adaptive process in the nervous system. Extensive research on alcohol has not yet been able to identify any adapting system (Goldstein, 1976; Kalant, 1987). In addition, the inconsistent relationship between tolerance and physical dependence remains unexplained.

Some investigators have opted to seek answers to the puzzle of tolerance by continuing the search for an alcohol-induced physiological adaptive reaction. Others have become less sanguine about this search and have begun to seek alternative explanations for alcohol tolerance and dependence. This latter approach has attracted the interest primarily of behavioral scientists. From time to time throughout this century, incidental observations and findings have been reported that appear logically inconsistent with the traditional pharmacological view of functional tolerance. During the last decade, systematic research on the effect of environmental factors upon the response to alcohol has accumulated. This additional evidence provides a more direct and explicit challenge to the assumption that tolerance and physical dependence upon alcohol can be explained solely by a central physiological homeostatic reaction to the pharmacological effects of the drug. Consequently, the nature of the adaptive process underlying alcohol tolerance and dependence has become increasingly controversial. This debate has wide ramifications because assumptions about the nature of alcohol tolerance inevitably carry practical social implications. Thus different notions about alcohol tolerance have also stimulated clashing perspectives on the risks of alcohol use and on the appropriate treatment for alcoholism (Peele, 1983).

## The Seeds of Doubt

Systematic research on the notion that alcohol tolerance is not completely governed by the pharmacological action and degree of exposure to the drug is comparatively recent. However, the idea itself has a long history. In 1919, Mellanby reported an interesting series of studies on the impairing effect of a dose of alcohol on the gait of dogs. He was primarily interested in determining threshold BACs for the onset and offset of impairment while plasma alcohol levels were rising and declining, respectively. His studies provided the first demonstration of acute tolerance, for he found the impairment evoked by a given BAC was more intense on the rising than on the declining limb of the BAC curve. Mellanby's important finding prompted much subsequent research on acute alcohol tolerance. Because this phenomenon occurs during the administration of a single dose, it has generally been perceived as irrelevant to chronic alcohol tolerance, which is assumed to require a history of repeated doses. However, it is not clear that Mellanby held this opinion. In discussing his findings, he reported that the degree of alcohol-induced impairment was greater if the dog was restrained until gait was tested. If it walked freely after alcohol was received, it was evidently more tolerant insofar as the impairment was less and did not appear until higher BACs were reached. Thus Mellanby warned investigators that behavioral tolerance to alcohol could be influenced by the test conditions.

Newman and Card (1937a, 1937b) rated the "degree of drunkenness" of dogs habituated to alcohol for 13 months. When the animals had BACs of 300–500 mg/100 ml, the habituated dogs were more tolerant than drug-naive dogs. After 7 months of abstinence, habituated dogs still showed tolerance at BACs of 300 mg/100 ml, but tolerance was no longer evident at higher BACs. These observations led Newman and Card to suggest that "psychomotor compensatory mechanisms" were involved in alcohol tolerance.

A similar notion was advanced by Goldberg (1943), who used many sensory and psychomotor tasks to investigate the effect of alcohol on alcoholics and social drinkers. He was interested in the *appearance* and *disappearance* thresholds for the drug effect on each task. These thresholds were measured by the rising BAC at which impairment was first observed, and the declining BAC when impairment was no longer evident. His study demonstrated that the occurrence and the intensity of acute tolerance varied with the type of task and drinker. Overall greater tolerance (i.e., higher thresholds on both limbs of the BAC curve) was displayed by the alcoholic group on every task. This research was among the first to provide adequate scientific evidence for incidental clinical observations and reports that alcoholics have an exceptionally high degree of tolerance to alcohol. The findings are consistent with the notion that tolerance increases with drug exposure, and are generally attributed to drug use. However, Goldberg himself was not so sure that a drug exposure explanation was completely adequate. His discussion of the results emphasized that the degree to which alcoholics and normals differed in tolerance depended upon the task. Less difference was obtained on tasks that were new to both groups, like subtraction and coding. In contrast, tasks measuring ataxia while walking or standing showed alcoholics to be much more tolerant than normals. Goldberg noted that these latter tasks were ones that alcoholics likely had previous experience performing under alcohol, and speculated that tolerance may result in part from learning "to compensate psychically for the influence of alcohol" (1943, p. 120).

Goldberg's research led him to suspect that two factors were involved in alcohol tolerance: a pharmacological effect of drug exposure and some sort of learning. However, his evidence of greater tolerance among alcoholics than among social drinkers appears to have encouraged the acceptance of a drug exposure explanation at the expense of a learning notion.

Until individuals are diagnosed as alcoholics, they are not distinguished from the general population of social drinkers. The factors responsible for converting a social drinker to an excessive, alcoholic drinker are not well understood. One explanation is implied in the assumption that more prolonged use of alcohol should result in greater tolerance. Because of growing tolerance, higher doses of alcohol may be required to achieve the original effect, and this in turn may lead to increased consumption of alcohol. From this perspective, social drinkers' tolerance should increase with years of drinking experience, and they should show a corresponding rise in their alcohol intake.

Research on the drinking habits and alcohol tolerance of social drinkers has not been designed specifically to test the prediction that alcohol consumption and tolerance increase as a function of years of social drinking. However, some interesting pertinent observations have been reported. Some time ago, Fillmore (1974) raised questions about the adequacy of the notion that alcohol consumption increases as a function of prolonged alcohol use. She conducted a longitudinal study of social drinkers to examine the quantity and frequency of drinking, and signs of problem drinking at two points in their lives: when they were aged 16–25 (time 1), and some 20 years later (time 2). Contrary to the notion that use of alcohol may increase with greater years of drug use, Fillmore observed a movement in the direction of *moderate* drinking and a shift toward nonproblem drinking over this period. The measure of problem drinking at time 1 was weakly correlated with an individual's problem drinking status 20 years later, but the correlation explained so little of the variation that Fillmore concluded the evidence was inconsistent with the notion of a progressive increase in alcohol consumption and risk of problem drinking with continued alcohol use. Fillmore's evidence also contradicted the assumption that high alcohol consumption during early stages of a drinking career should, with time, result in the use of even larger amounts of alcohol. She observed that problem drinking at time 2 was independent of quantity and frequency of drinking at time 1.

Fillmore's findings led her to speculate that the move toward moderation may somehow be related to aging. A similar trend has also been observed in some of our research examining the relationship between age and drinking habits in a cross-sectional national survey of Canadians ranging in age from 21 to 90 (Vogel-Sprott, 1983). The dose of alcohol (mg/kg body weight) that drinkers reported drinking per occasion showed the quantity *declined* linearly with age in men and women, and was unrelated to social or economic variables. In contrast, frequency of drinking was independent of age and varied with the social and economic characteristics of the drinkers. Thus the findings also suggest moderation occurs as a function of age, and this results specifically from a reduction in the *size* of the dose, not the frequency of drinking occasions. A recent report of a 20-year longitudinal survey of social drinkers (Leino, 1990) has also noted a trend toward decreased quantity consumed per occasion over time.

A smaller per-kg dose of alcohol generally yields a lower BAC. Therefore, it might be thought that a gradual reduction in dose as drinkers age means that older persons obtain lower BACs on social drinking occasions. However, the interpretation of the finding is complicated by the fact that the proportion of body water in weight also declines with age. Older persons have proportionally less body water per kg body weight. Thus the volume for distribution of alcohol becomes smaller with age, and the concentration of alcohol increases. As a result, the administration of a given mg/kg dose of alcohol is likely to generate higher peak BACs in older individuals. Confirmation of this effect has been provided by administering a fairly high intravenous dose of alcohol to humans (Vestal et al., 1977). In studies in our laboratory (Vogel-Sprott & Barrett, 1984) we have administered a moderate oral dose and observed older individuals to have higher BACs than younger social drinkers. Together the findings make it clear that a reduction in dose with age does not necessarily mean that lower BACs are occurring, but the interpretation is still unclear. Perhaps a reduction in consumption represents a type of self-titration to maintain BACs consistent with those a drinker obtained at a younger age. If this were the case, then maintaining the same BACs during one's drinking career would imply that an escalation of the BAC is not required to obtain the original desired effect of the drug. In other words, no tolerance develops. Yet this interpretation, too, is equivocal. In older drinkers, the reduced proportion of body water in body mass will raise the BAC resulting from a given dose. Thus, even if older drinkers lower their doses, they could still obtain equal or higher BACs than those customarily attained at an earlier age. If this were the case, then the development of tolerance would be implicated. Unfortunately, evidence that social drinkers' doses of alcohol diminish with age is not sufficient to tell us how alcohol tolerance may change with years of social drinking. Information on this question requires a longitudinal study of drinkers, or an experiment in which the effect of a given BAC is assessed in social drinkers who range widely in age.

Some of our early experiments tested alcohol tolerance as a function of years of social drinking (Newton, 1978; Vogel-Sprott & Barrett, 1984). In these studies, a moderate dose of alcohol was administered to social drinkers who ranged in age from 18 to 63. BACs were measured after drinking, and when a specific rising and declining BAC occurred, subjects performed tests of psychomotor performance, balance, and bead stringing. Under these conditions, the alcohol-induced impairment of each task intensified with the drinker's age. Although the subjects were tested when their BACs were identical, older individuals with some 30 to 40 years more drinking experience displayed *less* tolerance.

The drinking habit surveys and the laboratory measures of behavioral impairment were not specifically designed to test the assumption that alcohol tolerance and alcohol consumption both increase as a function of years of alcohol use. However, this notion seems difficult to reconcile with the evidence of these studies. The results should have shown that older social drinkers administer larger doses and are more tolerant to the effects of a given dose of alcohol. Yet the observations actually seem to suggest the reverse. Social drinkers appear to reduce their dose of alcohol as they become older, and they display less behavioral tolerance to a moderate dose of alcohol.

Observations gleaned from various studies that seem inconsistent with pharmacological explanations for the development of alcohol tolerance are useful because they suggest that there may still be some room for doubt. But an adequate challenge can only be provided by experiments designed to test and demonstrate the influence of other, nonpharmacological, factors on tolerance. A crucial control in such experiments is the provision of equivalent drug exposure to all subjects, so that the potential tolerance resulting from the pharmacological action of the drug is held constant. Under these conditions, another factor can be manipulated and its effect on tolerance can be assessed. The results of studies that adopted this strategy began to appear in the 1960s, and their findings are discussed in the next chapter.

# 2

## Nonpharmacological Factors Affecting Alcohol Tolerance

**N**onpharmacological variables refer to factors that can occur independently of the pharmacological action of a drug. Environmental circumstances under which a drug is administered or experienced are examples of nonpharmacological factors that have received considerable research attention.

One nonpharmacological factor, long suspected to affect behavioral tolerance to alcohol, is task practice under the drug. Mellanby (1919) initially suggested this possibility, and others later speculated that such practice resulted in learning to compensate for the effect of alcohol (Goldberg, 1943; Newman & Card, 1937a, 1937b). Interest in this longstanding suspicion appears to have been revived by Dews (1962), who suggested that a frequently intoxicated individual may acquire behavioral strategies that compensate for some impairing effects of alcohol. The first studies of the effect of task practice under alcohol appeared a few years later. These initial studies are particularly interesting because the observations were not questioned, but their interpretations were strenuously debated. The findings of these initial experiments, and the ensuing interpretive problems, make an interesting story.

### Early Studies

Initial experiments testing task practice effects on alcohol tolerance were conducted by Chen (1968, 1972). His studies involved two groups that practiced a task equally often, either *before* or *after* receiving equivalent doses of alcohol. In his first experiment, two groups of rats were trained to criterion on a temporal circular maze for food reward. The groups then received a 1.2 mg/kg dose of alcohol on each of 4 days. A "behavioral" group received alcohol *before* running the maze, and a "physiological" group received alcohol *after* running the maze. Tolerance was subsequently tested by administering alcohol to both groups prior to task performance. The alcohol-before group displayed significantly less behavioral disruption under alcohol (i.e., more tolerance) than did the alcohol-after group. That is, the behavioral group that had practiced the maze under alcohol was more tolerant to the disruptive effect of alcohol than was the physiological group with the same history of alcohol and maze exposure but with no experience performing the maze under alcohol.

An extension of the research by Chen (1972) tested the acquisition and the retention of tolerance induced by task practice under alcohol. Tolerance was tested at the conclusion of the practice phase of the study, and the retention of tolerance was tested after a 2-week drug-free rest. These tests demonstrated that the behavioral group, whose practice occurred under alcohol, was more tolerant, and their tolerance was well retained over the 2-week rest period. Chen noted that the relatively stable, long-lasting retention of behavioral tolerance resembled learning more than some physiological habituation process that should wax with exposure to alcohol and wane when it was withdrawn. This led Chen to conclude that learning, occurring during task practice under alcohol, must contribute to the development of tolerance.

Chen appears to be the first investigator to use a "before–after" design to manipulate task practice under alcohol while holding the amount of exposure to the drug constant for all subjects. This design has since been adopted to examine the development of alcohol tolerance during the performance of a variety of tasks (Chen, 1979; de Souza Moreira, Caprigliore, & Masur, 1981; LeBlanc, Kalant, & Gibbins, 1976; Mansfield, Benedict, & Woods, 1983). Although evidence from this research has been consistent with the phenomenon initially reported by Chen, his interpretation of the evidence has been controversial.

## Competing Interpretations

### Functional Demand

Some investigators completely rejected a learning interpretation of Chen's evidence. It was argued that performance under alcohol

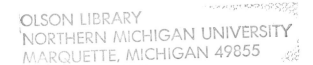

places greater demand on neuronal functioning, and greater neuronal activity hastens the physiological process of adaptation to drug effects (LeBlanc, Gibbins, & Kalant, 1973). This "functional demand" hypothesis proposed that the intoxicated practice required of the behavioral group in Chen's research simply accelerated the rate of physiological adaptation to alcohol and involved no learning. All groups would eventually display tolerance. It merely developed more quickly with the greater functional demand posed by intoxicated practice. This proposal led to studies that extended the alcohol treatment to 24 days, and compared the effect of daily intoxicated task practice to the effect of physiological exposure to the same daily doses of alcohol (LeBlanc et al., 1976). The tolerance of the physiological group in this research was assessed by testing task performance under alcohol six times, at 4-day intervals during the 24 days of drug treatment. After the treatment, the tolerance of the groups was compared when they performed the task under a dose of alcohol. This test showed the tolerance of the physiological and the behavioral groups did not differ. Thus the authors concluded that learning through task practice under alcohol was not necessary for the development of tolerance. Intoxicated practice just hastened the process of biological adaptation to alcohol and added nothing to the ultimate degree of tolerance observed. But this interpretation was also challenged.

Wenger, Berlin, and Woods (1980), and Wenger et al. (1981) pointed out that a physiological drug exposure group having tolerance tests at 4-day intervals essentially receives intermittent task practice under alcohol, and this provides an opportunity for learning. Wenger et al. (1980, 1981) demonstrated that groups receiving drugged task practice (daily or intermittently) became tolerant, whereas a physiological control group receiving only one tolerance test on the final day of the experiment displayed no tolerance. Therefore, these investigators concluded that an animal must perform the task under drug to become tolerant and argued that their evidence clearly implicated learning factors in tolerance.

The disagreement over whether learning was responsible for Chen's findings appeared to be resolved in favor of learning. But the controversy was not over. Those who favored a learning explanation entered the debate and proposed different interpretations of the sort of learning that was involved. Chen had argued that task practice enhanced tolerance by allowing the learning of a behavioral strategy to compensate for the impairing effect of alcohol. This view was consistent with the earlier notions about tolerance to the behavioral effects of a drug (Dews, 1962; Goldberg, 1943; Newman & Card,

1937a, 1937b). However, more recent learning research with drugs led to divergent interpretations of the learning process involved in experiments using a before–after design.

## Drug State Dependent Learning

Investigations of transfer of training on a task from one situation to another indicate that more transfer (i.e., better performance of a task) is obtained if stimulus events during training and transfer are identical. Drug state dependent learning (SDL) is specifically concerned with the drug state of the subject during training and transfer tests. If a task is learned while a subject is under the influence of a central acting drug, subsequent performance of the task is better under the drug and poorer without the drug. Similarly, subjects trained in an undrugged state perform more poorly if subsequent tests are conducted under drug. Reviews of SDL (Overton, 1972, 1984) have suggested the findings indicate that the memory of a learned response depends upon the existence of a similar drug state during initial learning and the subsequent test of retrieval.

It has been suggested that alcoholic "blackouts" are examples of SDL, because the drinker in a subsequently sober state has no memory of events or activities occurring during the drinking episode (Goodwin, 1971; Goodwin, Othmer, Halikas, & Freemon, 1970; Mayfield & Montgomery, 1972). These clinical observations are analogous to SDL effects obtained by training under drug and subsequently testing drug-free. Research has provided a demonstration of SDL effects with alcohol (Goodwin, Powell, Bremer, Hoine, & Stern, 1969; Overton, 1972). SDL has usually been investigated in a $2 \times 2$ experimental design that involves four groups. Two groups are initially trained on a task under drug (D), and two receive training with no drug (N). Subsequent tests of retention under drug (D) or no drug (N) are crossed with each training condition. The treatment groups trained with or without drug and tested drug-free may be designated, respectively, as DN and NN. The remaining two groups, DD and ND, represent those with different training histories tested for retention under the drug.

Such studies are of particular interest because they include two groups, DD and ND, that practice under drug or drug-free and are subsequently tested under drug. This is the procedure used in Chen's before-after experiments to show the tolerance-inducing effect of task practice under alcohol. In both instances, the procedure yields similar findings: When tested under alcohol, the group that had training under the drug displays better performance than the group whose training occurred in a drug-free state. A carry-over effect of training to subsequent performance implies learning, and the consistent results of the procedure in studies with different orientations adds important support for the assumption that the effects are due to learning.

But what is it that is being learned? SDL assumes that what is learned is identical whether the subject is under drug or drug-free, and emphasizes memory retrieval. Changes in the drug state are considered to have amnesic effects, so that what was learned could not be remembered as well. In contrast, Chen suspected that some new compensatory response strategy was learned by performing a task under drug, and this learning opportunity was absent when the task was practiced in a drug-free state. From Chen's perspective, subjects with drug-free training show poorer subsequent performance under alcohol because of a learning deficit. They have no pertinent learned behavior to remember.

Many reasons may be offered for preferring a memory or an adaptive learned response explanation of what appears to be the same evidence. However, it may not be necessary to choose between the two interpretations, because there is an important difference between studies using a before–after design and those investigating SDL. Although both types of experiments provide training on a task with or without drug, this training begins at different stages of familiarity with the task. SDL studies administer drugged training *while* a new task is being learned, when memory is presumably being consolidated. In contrast, before-after studies begin drugged training *after* a task is learned, when drug-free performance has reached a criterion of proficiency and memory of the requisite task responses may be established. It may be that a developing memory of newly acquired task responses is impaired by changes in drug state. However, after a task is mastered, the memory needed for performance is likely to have developed, and retrieval of this memory may be little influenced by changes in drug state. It is possible that when a task is well learned, subsequent training under drug provides an opportunity to learn some new response strategies that adapt performance to the new drugged condition.

The interpretation of before–after design studies in terms of memory or new learned responses remains open. But these are not the only possible learning interpretations of the findings. A Pavlovian conditioning theory of drug tolerance offers another alternative (Hinson & Siegel, 1980; Siegel, 1976, 1978).

## Pavlovian Conditioning

This learning interpretation of drug tolerance assumes that the administration of the dose of a drug has a *constant* effect that evokes a *drug-like* response, resembling pharmacologically induced disturbances. This disturbance, in turn, may elicit a reflexive compensatory reaction that is opposite in direction to the drug effect. This *drug-opposite compensatory reaction* serves to counteract the disturbance and maintain homeostasis, and may *increase* in strength when the drug is readministered. Thus this compensatory reaction could have an adaptive value, minimizing the magnitude and duration of a drug effect.

The pharmacological interpretation of tolerance also assumes that a drug-opposite compensatory reaction is evoked by a drug. The new contribution of conditioning theory is that repeated drug administrations represent learning trials that result in an anticipatory conditioned drug-compensatory reaction to environmental events that predict the administration of a drug. In this analysis, a *conditional stimulus (CS)* refers to an event (i.e., drug administration ritual and environmental context) associated with the occurrence of a drug. Such a predictive stimulus serves as a cue for drug. An *unconditional stimulus (US)* is the actual pharmacological stimulation of a drug that elicits an *unconditioned response (UR)*. The UR is assumed to evoke a drug-like and a drug-opposite compensatory reaction. This relationship is illustrated below, where the events are shown by conventional classical conditioning terms and by alternative symbols that will be used when our theoretical analysis is presented in Chapter 4.

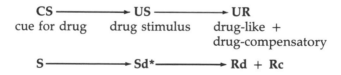

$$CS \longrightarrow US \longrightarrow UR$$
$$\text{cue for drug} \quad \text{drug stimulus} \quad \text{drug-like } +$$
$$\text{drug-compensatory}$$
$$S \longrightarrow Sd^* \longrightarrow Rd + Rc$$

The development of drug tolerance is viewed as the net effect of the drug-like response, plus a compensatory response that grows with repeated administrations of a drug and opposes the drug effect. Repetitions of the drug that involve CS-US pairings are considered to permit the CS-US association to be learned, so that the environmental cue for drug comes to serve as a predictive signal for the drug stimulus. When tolerance is established under these conditions, conditioning theory predicts that the predrug cue evokes a *conditioned compensatory reaction (CR)* that counteracts the drug effect. Tolerance arising in a classical conditioning paradigm is depicted as:

**CS** ———————————➤ **CR**
cue for drug      conditioned compensatory reaction

Such a relationship could also be symbolized as:

**S** ——————————➤ **Rc**

An experimental design, termed "discriminative control of tolerance," was devised to test conditioned morphine tolerance (Siegel, 1979). This design has since been used in studies of many drugs, including alcohol. The method essentially involves two groups of subjects that both receive the same repeated dose of a drug and of a *placebo*, that is, an inert substance. The groups differ only with respect to the environmental setting associated with the receipt of each substance. For example, one group could receive the drug in a bright, noisy room (environment A) and the inert substance in a dark, quiet room (environment B). For purposes of control, the relationship between the environments and the substance administered would be reversed for the second group. In our example, the second group would receive the drug in environment B and the inert substance in environment A. Under this training regimen, equivalent doses of the drug and of the inert substance are administered to all subjects, equally often at the same intervals. The two groups also have the same opportunity to associate the drug stimulus with a distinctive environmental stimulus. The only difference between the groups is the environmental cue (A or B) that predicts the drug. Conditioning theory predicts that when tolerance is established under these conditions, the amount of tolerance displayed depends upon the presence or absence of the environmental cue predicting the drug. Subjects should display more tolerance when the drug is administered in the context of cues previously paired with the pharmacological stimulation, and less or none when the drug is administered in the presence of cues that have not been associated with the receipt of the drug. In other words, maximal tolerance should be displayed by the subjects of each group when the drug is expected, and least when the drug is unexpected.

Drug tolerance is assumed to reflect the combined effect of a drug-like and a drug-opposite reaction. Because a drug must be administered to test tolerance, it is not possible to obtain a direct observation of the compensatory reaction uncontaminated by the drug effect. However, the theory of conditioned tolerance indicates that tests to demonstrate a conditioned compensatory reaction can be performed by administering a placebo to tolerant subjects in the context of cues previously associated with the receipt of the drug. In this case, conditioning theory predicts a stronger drug-opposite response to placebo in the presence of drug-associated cues, and little or no such reaction when these cues are absent.

Reviews of studies testing a Pavlovian conditioning interpretation of drug tolerance find considerable support for the model (e.g., Hinson & Siegel, 1980; Siegel, 1989). Experiments have investigated conditioned tolerance to the hypothermic effect of alcohol in rats (Cappell, Roach, & Poulos, 1981; Crowell, Hinson, & Siegel, 1981; Le, Poulos & Cappell, 1979; Mansfield & Cunningham, 1980; Siegel & Sdao-Jarvie, 1986). Other experiments with humans have investigated heart rate and cognitive task performance (Dafters & Anderson, 1982; Newlin, 1986; Shapiro & Nathan, 1986; Staiger & White, 1988). The results of these studies are in general agreement. "Expected" groups (i.e., those who receive alcohol in the familiar drug-associated environment) display greater tolerance than the "unexpected" groups, whose alcohol is administered in a novel environment. In addition, the receipt of a placebo has often resulted in a stronger drug-opposite compensatory response when it is administered in the presence of predictive cues for alcohol. These effects are not readily explained by a traditional pharmacological view that assumes tolerance depends solely upon the systemic effect of alcohol exposure. But they are consistent with the conditioning model of tolerance that emphasizes a learned stimulus expectancy for drug, in response to the presence of cues that have reliably predicted the administration of alcohol.

Pavlovian conditioning has been offered as an explanation for the tolerance-enhancing effect of task practice under alcohol obtained in studies using a before–after design. Hinson and Siegel (1980) have pointed out that a before–after design creates different relationships between predrug cues and the administration of alcohol for each group of subjects. For example, the behavioral group in Chen's experiment (1968) had an opportunity to learn to expect alcohol in the presence of the task because it was consistently associated with drug effects during all practice sessions. Thus the task was part of the environmental cues that could have come to signal drug effects and to evoke a conditioned drug-compensatory response that would be observed as tolerance. In contrast, the physiological group had no opportunity to associate the task with the drug because they performed the task and then received the drug later in another room.

Because the subsequent tolerance test involved administering alcohol in the task environment, this unique situation for the physiological group could explain its lack of tolerance. Therefore, tolerance, ostensibly resulting from the acquisition of a behavioral strategy to compensate for the effects of the drug, may have resulted from learned stimulus expectancy for drug.

## Too Many Explanations?

Classically conditioned cues for a drug have been found to influence tolerance to alcohol and many other drugs, such as opiates (Siegel, 1975, 1976, 1977, 1978, 1979), barbiturates (Hinson, Poulos, & Cappell, 1982; Hinson & Siegel, 1986), cocaine (Hinson & Poulos, 1981), and the neuroleptic haloperidol (Poulos & Hinson, 1982). These results have fostered some recognition that traditional pharmacological explanations of alcohol tolerance may have to be expanded to consider environmental–neurochemical interactions (Kalant & Khanna, 1980), but these investigators still consider the issue to be one of understanding how cellular or other biological adaptive changes are initiated by alcohol. Environmental variables are seen as qualifying factors that modify the ability of the drug to induce a compensatory reaction. This orientation has led to valuable insights on neurotransmitters and neuropeptides that affect the acquisition and retention of learned behavior. Moreover, manipulations of these neurochemicals have been found to have similar effects on the acquisition and retention of alcohol tolerance (e.g., Frankel, Khanna, Kalant, & LeBlanc, 1978; Hoffman, Ritzmann, Walter, & Tabakoff, 1978; Le, Khanna, Kalant, & LeBlanc, 1981; Speisky & Kalant, 1985). Thus it seems that learning is at least as important as the drug action in determining tolerance.

A Pavlovian conditioning interpretation of tolerance has stimulated the accumulation of considerable evidence implicating learning. Possibly for this reason, the most favored learning interpretation of the tolerance resulting from task practice in before–after design experiments is that of classical conditioning. Nonetheless, the results of before–after design studies are logically still open to all of the various competing interpretations. The behavioral group, which typically shows most tolerance, also experiences greater demands on behavioral functioning under alcohol. Therefore, the functional demand hypothesis cannot be unequivocally dismissed. Even if the tolerance displayed by the behavioral group is attributed to learning, the interpretation remains equivocal because either classical conditioning or state dependent learning could explain the results. In retrospect, it seems that a before–after design provides remarkably consistent evidence but simultaneously clouds its interpretation.

The debate over the interpretation of the results of before–after design studies gave no serious consideration to the original hypothesis that led Chen to use the experimental design. This neglect may explain why no one pointed out that a before–after design could not adequately test Chen's notion that the tolerance resulting from drugged task practice reflects the acquisition of some new response strategy to compensate for the effect of alcohol. A *strategy* commonly refers to learned behavior that is displayed whenever warranted by the circumstances. Unless the behavior yields some desirable outcome, it is unlikely to occur. Now suppose Chen is correct, and some new drug-compensatory response is being learned during drugged practice. Its occurrence also should be determined by its consequence. This sort of evidence cannot be provided in a before–after design study because only one group receives drugged task practice, so that the effect on tolerance of manipulating the consequence of performance cannot be evaluated. It may be that task practice under alcohol provides an opportunity to learn a new compensatory response, but its display depends upon the consequence of this response. This sort of evidence would support Chen's hypothesis, but it cannot be derived from his before–after design studies.

It seems ironic that Chen's data on the effect of task practice on alcohol tolerance attracted so much attention, but that his hypothesis generated so little consideration. The emergence of different interpretations of the data may have sidetracked interest in his hypothesis to some extent. But investigators disposed to consider the possibility that learning affects drug tolerance may have also considered Chen's notion implausible and difficult to test. Unlike Pavlovian conditioning theory, which specified the factors governing the learning of stimulus expectancy for drug, there appeared to be no theoretical framework for testing predictions about the sort of learning Chen was discussing. In addition, the implications of his hypothesis appeared to conflict with those of classically conditioned tolerance. Chen's notion implied that tolerance is affected by learning about events that occur *after* the administration of alcohol, whereas conditioning theory considers tolerance to require repeated drug exposures that permit learning about events that occur before the administration of the drug.

In summary, there has been little interest in the idea that alcohol tolerance can be influenced by learning after alcohol has been received. Nonetheless, other incidental observations and research evidence during the 1960s and 1970s hinted that earlier investigators were on the right track. Moreover, the evidence reviewed in the next chapter shows that neither the biological action of alcohol nor classical conditioning provided a complete account of alcohol tolerance. A more adequate explanation will require consideration of the learned consequences of behavior *after* the drug is received.

# 3

## The Plot Thickens: Tolerance and Events after Drinking

Folklore and anecdotes are no substitutes for scientific evidence, but they sometimes prompt a curiosity that may lead to hypotheses. Stories about drinking escapades are a case in point. It is quite common for drinkers to describe the experience of suddenly sobering up during some emergency. Embellishments of this situation also occur in jokes. "Did you hear about the alcoholic who was dead drunk in the attic when fire broke out? He ran down the stairs and turned on the alarm!" The interesting feature of these anecdotes and jokes is their common underlying theme. They all imply that behavioral tolerance to alcohol is affected by events after drinking has occurred. The idea that a drinker can "turn on" tolerance when needed has never been given serious consideration. Nonetheless, much folklore describes situations in which an intoxicated individual appears deliberately able to compensate for the disrupting effects of alcohol *when the consequences of tolerance are advantageous.*

The display of tolerance when it yields a desirable consequence was also reported by Goldberg and Havard (1968), who described the development of technology to determine blood alcohol concentration (BAC) from breath samples. Before such tests were available, a medical examination of suspected impaired drivers was required to support the charge. These clinical assessments of suspects proved

unreliable and insensitive as a method of detecting alcohol impairment. . . . Suspects faced with an examination by a doctor called in

by the police are often able to pull themselves together sufficiently
to pass clinical tests as a result of the physiological and psychological "alarm" reaction induced by the crisis in which they find
themselves. Indeed, it is not unknown for a driver to satisfy the
police surgeon only to have to be assisted from the police station
after the crisis has passed and the symptoms of intoxication have
reasserted themselves. (Goldberg & Havard, 1968, p. 8)

This report also describes a comparatively sudden, on–off display
of alcohol tolerance that seems clearly to be related to environmental
events occurring after alcohol has been administered. Such stories are
amusing probably because they seem implausible and violate the
usual notion of drug tolerance as a chronic and fairly stable individual
characteristic that develops gradually because of drug use. In view of
the research on Pavlovian conditioning of tolerance, it might now be
conceded that some variation in a drinker's display of tolerance may
occur as a result of changes in the environmental cues that predict the
administration of alcohol. But conditioning theory is exclusively
concerned with the expectation of receiving a drug, created by
stimulus events associated with the presentation of a drug. The
questions of how, why, or whether alcohol tolerance is affected by
events after the drug has been received, remain unanswered.

## Clues from Studies Using Within-Subjects Designs

Studies of drug tolerance using Pavlovian conditioning procedures
typically do not address the possibility that tolerance is affected by
events occurring *after* a drug is received. Such information is more
likely to be gleaned by observing the effect of a drug on the
performance of a single subject when events during the drugged
behavior are changed. Technically speaking, we are looking for
evidence on tolerance obtained in studies using a *within-subjects*
design. Such a design is more commonly used in learning studies in
which a subject's response on some task is related to some important
consequence. This form of training is referred to, variously, as *operant
conditioning* or *instrumental learning*. In this training paradigm, the
experimenter controls the environmental consequence of a subject's
behavior. For example, some favorable event, like food to a hungry
rat, may be contingent upon the display of a particular response, such
as a bar press. Instrumental and operant learning experiments often
refer to the consequence as *reinforcement,* and a favorable consequence
would be termed a *positive reinforcer.* The training involves the

administration of a consequence according to some rule, or *schedule*. In our example, one food pellet for one bar press would be an example of a simple schedule, but many different schedules are possible. For example, a fixed interval (FI) schedule would administer one food pellet for a response per a specific interval, regardless of how many bar presses were displayed. A differential low rate of reinforcement (DRL) is a more complex schedule in which a food pellet would only be administered for a bar press if the subject delays the response for a specified time. If the schedule is always the same whenever the subject performs the task, the training is said to occur under a *single* schedule of reinforcement.

To compare the effect of different reinforcement schedules on a subject's behavior, some experiments use more than one reinforcement schedule. This is referred to as *multiple* schedules of reinforcement. A simple example would involve two different schedules, each in effect for a time and alternating while the subject performs the task. More detailed descriptions of single and multiple schedules of reinforcement and their effects on behavior are provided in learning texts (e.g., Schwartz, 1978).

Many studies have used a within-subjects design to investigate the development of drug tolerance under multiple schedules of reinforcement. The results of these experiments are of particular interest because they could provide some information concerning the suspicion that tolerance is affected by events after a drug is received. The findings of such studies also provide a particularly good hunting ground for clues because a subject performs the same task under the same drug state. Thus the experimental design provides a control for the effects of expecting the drug, the drug state, and functional demands on performance. These are the important factors that have been implicated in other research on tolerance, so it is important to understand exactly how their control is achieved.

A within-subjects design in which a drug is repeatedly administered to a subject who performs under multiple schedules of reinforcement will allow the subject to acquire a stimulus expectancy for the drug. This is because the administration of repeated doses of a drug could be associated with events that may come to signal the receipt of the drug. Although the degree to which a subject learns to expect the drug may affect the tolerance displayed, the events determining the expectancy *precede* the administration of a drug and do not involve events *after* the drug is received. Thus the influence of expecting the drug should remain constant despite subsequent events that occur during performance under a drug. In other words, the events predicting the administration of a drug are different and can be independent of events predicting the consequences. Because a subject performs the same task under the drug throughout the course of the experiment, the functional demands on performance are unchanged and there is no change in a subject's drug state. Thus no variation in functional demand or drug state could affect performance under the drug. Within-subjects experiments examining the effect of multiple schedules of reinforcement on tolerance only manipulate environmental consequences of performance *after* a drug has been administered. Thus, if the tolerance displayed by a subject varies when the reinforcement schedule changes, it must be attributed to the manipulation of the environmental consequence of performance under drug.

An early example of such research was provided by Schuster, Dockens, and Woods (1966), who trained rats to bar press for food under alternating FI and DRL reinforcement schedules, with a light signaling a change in the schedule. After drug-free baseline training ensured a stable pattern of performance by an animal under each schedule, a dose of *d*-amphetamine was administered before each bar pressing session. The stimulating effect of the dose initially increased the response rate under both schedules. After 30 days of treatment, tolerance to the behavioral effects of *d*-amphetamine was observed under the DRL schedule. But the high response rate initially induced by amphetamine showed no decrease when the FI schedule was in effect. Thus tolerance was absent during the FI schedule and present during the DRL schedule. This "on–off" display of tolerance by the same animal under alternating reinforcement schedules bears a striking resemblance to the behavior of the intoxicated suspect in our impaired driving story. Schuster et al. (1966) also speculated that the effects were determined by the events during drugged performance. They noted that the initial stimulant effect of the drug disrupted performance so that food was lost under the DRL schedule, but not under the FI schedule.

The effect of the response–reinforcement relationship on tolerance was further examined (Schuster et al., 1966) using a task in which a signal predicted an electric shock that could be avoided if the animals ran when the signal was presented. The stimulating effect of *d*-amphetamine increased avoidance responses and resulted in fewer shocks being received. Although *d*-amphetamine was administered for 35 days, tolerance to the stimulating effect failed to develop in any rat during this period. In discussing these findings, Schuster et al. noted that the initial effect of *d*-amphetamine on the avoidance response did not reduce the reward (i.e., shock avoidance). Thus they suggested that tolerance may be governed by a *loss of reinforcement* principle. They proposed that behavioral tolerance develops when the drug effect disrupts the performance required to obtain positive reinforcement. Conversely, when the behavioral effect of a drug either enhances or does not change the density of reinforcement, tolerance may not be observed.

The loss of reinforcement hypothesis provided the first step in calling attention to the importance of the consequence of performance under a drug. Many ensuing studies using multiple reinforcement schedules have confirmed that the drug tolerance a subject displays is affected by the reinforcement schedule during drugged performance (e.g., Branch, 1983; Brocco, Rastogi, & McMillan, 1983; Elsmore, 1976; Galbicka, Lee, & Branch, 1980). However, the findings have not consistently supported a loss of reinforcement principle (Corfield-Sumner & Stolerman, 1978). The hypothesis often runs into difficulty because a particular reinforcement schedule that induces behavioral tolerance to a drug in one situation may fail to do so in another (Ferraro & Grilly, 1973). Nonetheless, the research has made a valuable contribution to the documentation and description of variations in drug tolerance under different reinforcement schedules. Moreover, these findings have been obtained with many different types of drugs. The results are clearly inconsistent with the assumption that some central drug-induced physiological adaptation accounts for tolerance. However, the impact of the evidence is constrained because the research offers no conceptual framework to account for the influence of reinforcement schedules on tolerance (Branch, 1984).

## Suspicions Concerning the Consequences of Tolerance

The reason for the intermittent success of the loss of reinforcement principle to predict drug tolerance remains an open question. Many speculations about this problem have been offered, but one by Ferraro and Grilly (1973) is particularly interesting. They found that monkeys failed to develop tolerance to a drug under a reinforcement schedule that had induced tolerance in other types of animals. In puzzling over their results, they suggested that the restraining device needed to ensure that the monkeys remained seated before the task may have impeded the ability of the animals to adjust their performance to compensate for the effect of the drug. They speculated that a failure to display tolerance might occur in situations that constrain behavior so that no drug-compensatory response can be made. This notion implies that tolerance requires some task-specific compensatory response and bears a remarkable similarity to Chen's (1968, 1972) proposal that behavioral tolerance involves some new behavioral strategy to compensate for the effect of a drug on task performance. Yet the research by Schuster et al. (1966) additionally suggested that the reinforcement of performance under a drug is also important.

These ideas led to the hypothesis that has provided the major impetus for our research: *A crucial factor governing behavioral tolerance is the consequence of displaying a compensatory response.* To induce tolerance, some desirable consequence must be associated with the display of drug-compensatory performance, so that compensating for the drug effect yields the most favorable consequence. This hypothesis predicts behavioral tolerance by what is *gained* by a compensatory response. This is different from a loss of reinforcement hypothesis, which attributed tolerance to the loss of reward occasioned by the *transition* from drug-free to drugged performance, and did not consider the drug-compensatory response. However, both hypotheses assume that the occurrence of a response can be predicted by its consequence, and the response that yields the most desirable outcome is most likely to be displayed. The application of these assumptions to drug-compensatory performance to predict drug tolerance is the novel feature of our hypothesis.

Our views prompted a retrospective look at the results of one of our early studies examining alcohol tolerance in male social drinkers (Vogel-Sprott, 1979). This research used a within-subjects design where each subject was trained on a paper-and-pencil coding task, and a pursuit rotor task that required accurate tracking of a rotating target. One trial on each task lasted 3 minutes. Coding and pursuit rotor performance were assessed, respectively, by the number of items correctly coded, and the time on target. After drug-free baseline training, four weekly drinking sessions were administered. During these sessions, experimental subjects received alcohol, and controls received a nonalcoholic drink. All subjects were treated alike in every other way, and every subject performed both tasks equally often after drinking during each session. The performance of the two tasks by the control group did not change significantly during these sessions. This was no surprise: They had received no alcohol, and the subjects had been well trained in the two tasks before drinking sessions began. It is the results of the group receiving alcohol that are of interest. They displayed impaired performance on both tasks during the first drinking session. On the subsequent three sessions, the development of tolerance was increasingly evident, but only when the subject performed the coding task. The initial alcohol-induced impairment of pursuit rotor performance showed no reduction, even though a subject performed the two tasks within minutes of each other on every drinking session. This differential on–off display of alcohol tolerance by a subject was quite dramatic, although it had not been predicted and the study was not designed to identify the factor responsible for these results.

Although the coding and pursuit rotor tasks differed on many dimensions, the notion that the outcome of drug-compensatory performance may affect tolerance led to a reexamination of this aspect of the tasks. It seemed possible that their consequences did differ in a fashion that might explain the findings. The coding task could have conveyed information to a subject about the adequacy of his performance because he could see the work completed on each trial. Such information, often called knowledge of results, or feedback, is found to operate like positive reinforcement and enhances the performance of humans (Schwartz & Lacey, 1982). In contrast, the pursuit rotor appeared to provide no such information. When subjects performed the pursuit rotor, they were not told their trial scores, and they could not accurately estimate their scores from one trial to the next. Thus we wondered if the presence of a desirable outcome for drug-compensatory performance may have been the factor responsible for the development of tolerance on the coding task. Could it be that tolerance failed to develop on the pursuit rotor task because there was no desirable consequence of drug-compensatory performance?

## Summary

The results of some within-subjects design studies do seem consistent with the hypothesis that drug tolerance is affected by its consequence. However, the findings described up to this point are only circumstantial because none of the experiments was specifically designed to test the hypothesis. Although past evidence seems to suggest that tolerance can be influenced by learning about events after a drug is administered, interest in the phenomenon has been overshadowed by a Pavlovian conditioning theory of tolerance that concerns events preceding the administration of a drug.

In retrospect, the domination of a classical conditioning explanation of drug tolerance is quite understandable. The well-established principles of Pavlovian conditioning provided a clear beacon to guide and stimulate research to obtain a coherent body of evidence on learned tolerance. Moreover, this approach could be readily incorporated within traditional notions of functional tolerance, where tolerance is assumed to develop gradually with accumulating drug exposures. Conditioning theory added a new feature to functional tolerance by demonstrating the importance of learning about events predicting the administration of a drug. But repeated drug exposures were still assumed to be required to strengthen a drug-compensatory reaction. Thus the theory of conditioned drug tolerance expands, but does not challenge, traditional assumptions.

In contrast, the hypothesis that learning about events *after* a drug has been received would seem less feasible. First, no theory had been suggested that might explain or predict this effect, and research without any conceptual framework is a bit like sailing through uncharted waters without a compass. Second, the hypothesis seemed to imply a learning process in the development of tolerance that has some volitional properties independent of the action of the drug. Such a proposal was clearly at odds with the traditional notion of tolerance induced by the action of a drug. The weight of prevailing opinion may have led experimenters to conclude the hypothesis was too implausible to merit attention, especially in the absence of any testable theory to guide the investigation.

Yet the neglect of this hypothesis has been a major oversight in efforts to understand alcohol tolerance in humans. Factors contributing to social drinkers' tolerance to alcohol are not understood. Although little credence has been given to the notion that events after drinking can affect alcohol tolerance, many events and activities commonly do occur after social drinking. Indeed, such situations are so ubiquitous that they are scarcely given any thought. Thus, if learning under such circumstances does affect tolerance, it could be an important pervasive determinant of social drinkers' tolerance. An impediment to the systematic investigation of this possibility has been the lack of some guiding theoretical framework. Pavlovian conditioning offered a valuable account of learned tolerance based upon events preceding the administration of a drug. But an expanded theory is needed to account for the acquisition of tolerance as a function of events occurring *before* and *after* a drug is received. The next chapter presents a theoretical model of learning that serves this purpose.

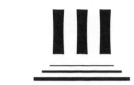

# LEARNING, EXPECTANCY, AND DRUG TOLERANCE

# 4

# *Theory Development*

The previous chapter examined clues suggesting that events during behavior under alcohol may affect tolerance. An examination of the evidence suggested that the association between a particular pair of events, a drug-compensatory response and its consequence, may be crucial. We also noted that the effect of this relationship may be analogous to learning under instrumental training, where the association between a response (R) and some important event (S*) is manipulated. However, adequate tests of such an hypothesis had not been performed, and no theory of tolerance incorporating an instrumental learning component had been proposed.

This chapter proposes a theory of learned tolerance that considers the contribution of events associated with the administration of a drug, *and* events associated with performance after a drug is received. Thus the theory proposes an account of tolerance that encompasses the effects of Pavlovian conditioning *and* instrumental learning. Pavlovian conditioning involves the pairing of some neutral stimulus (S) with another important stimulus (S*). The asterisk denotes an event that has some importance to a subject. Instrumental training pairs a different set of events: a response (R) and some important stimulus event (S*). During the first half of this century, the two procedures were viewed as completely different learning processes. Such a view, of course, would discourage any effort to develop a theory of learned tolerance that incorporated effects of classical conditioning and instrumental training. However, developments in learning theory suggest that the learning occurring under

45

the two training procedures is not necessarily independent. A review of these contemporary views of learning shows how they guided the development of our theory of learned tolerance.

## Contemporary Learning Theory

As research on learning has continued, earlier views of learning in terms of an association between a pair of stimuli (S-S*), or a response and a stimulus (R-S*), have expanded in favor of viewing learning in terms of an association between *any* pair of events (Bolles, 1979; Thompson & Voss, 1972). Essentially, the idea is that there could be four types of associations. They can be classified by whether a stimulus (S) or a response (R) is the first or second event in the relationship. These are illustrated in Figure 2. The rows identify the antecedent event, which could be either an environmental stimulus or a response. The columns identify the consequent event that also may be a stimulus or a response. The four cells within the matrix depict each class of association. To date, the findings on behavioral tolerance to drugs have only implicated the S-S association in the first row of the first column. Our theory of tolerance considers the two associations, S-S and R-S, in both rows of the first column. Thus our theory aims to expand explanations of learned tolerance beyond the current limits of the S-S associations involved in Pavlovian conditioning. Such an expansion, of course, would still be narrow in terms of providing a completely adequate theory of learning effects in tolerance. Consideration would have to be given to the associations shown in the second column of Figure 2.[1] The topic of a more comprehensive learning theory of tolerance is considered in Section VI, when we discuss some implications of our research.

The last few decades have produced a shift in learning theory, from a mechanical toward a cognitive interpretation (Bolles, 1979; Hall, 1982; Schwartz, 1978; Schwartz & Lacey, 1982). This development was fostered, in part, by many studies that showed learning could occur in the absence of any overt response. Pavlovian conditioning studies have shown that simply pairing a neutral stimulus with an important stimulus event that evokes a response cannot guarantee the development of a conditioned response. When two different neutral stimuli precede an important event, a conditioned response only develops to the first neutral stimulus, even though the

---

[1]S-R and R-R associations are termed "response expectancies" by Kirsch (1985), and are defined as expectancies of the occurrence of nonvolitional responses.

**ANTECEDENT**      **CONSEQUENT**

|  | Stimulus (S) | Response (R) |
|---|---|---|
| **Stimulus (S)** | S-S | S-R |
| **Response (R)** | R-S | R-R |

**FIGURE 2.** Possible associations between any combination of stimulus (S) and response (R) events.

second stimulus is closer in time to the important event. In this case, it appears that the first stimulus reliably signals the occurrence of the important event and makes the second signal redundant. Such findings have led to the proposal that learning under Pavlovian conditioning takes place only when a stimulus is informative and reliably predicts the occurrence or nonoccurrence of an important stimulus event (Egger & Miller, 1962; Kamin, 1969; Rescorla & Wagner, 1972; Wagner & Rescorla, 1972). Reviewers of instrumental and classical conditioning in humans have also argued that learning represents the acquisition of information through prior experience, instruction, or observation of event contingencies (Boakes, 1989; Brewer, 1974). Although the fundamental nature of the learning process is not settled, many theories now assume that learning consists of acquiring information about the predictable relationships between events.

Although the training procedures used in instrumental and Pavlovian conditioning are different, research now suggests that instrumental training can simultaneously involve classical conditioning. A simple illustration of this is provided by considering an animal in a Skinner box, where the presentation of a food pellet is contingent upon an animal's bar press and may be said to reward or reinforce the response. However, the situation also can be viewed in terms of a Pavlovian conditioning paradigm because the pellet could be identified as an important stimulus that evokes responses such as salivation. Because the neutral stimuli of the Skinner box are always present before the pellet is received, the box signals the pellet and may come to evoke a conditioned salivary response. In other words, whenever instrumental training is conducted, classical conditioning can occur simultaneously.

In the past, instrumental and Pavlovian conditioning procedures were distinguished by the type of responses that were trained.

Instrumental training involved voluntary responses, whereas Pavlovian conditioning applied to reflexive reactions. This distinction too has become blurred, as some evidence suggests that the same response can be trained by each procedure. For example, salivation can be a reflexive response to food, and Pavlovian conditioning experiments can reliably develop a classically conditioned salivary response. However, instrumental learning experiments show that the salivary response can be controlled by its consequences. Water-deprived animals may be trained to display high or low rates of salivation for water (Miller & Carmona, 1967). It seems that instrumental learning and classical conditioning may each affect the same response.

Interactions between Pavlovian and instrumental training procedures are described in many learning texts (Hall, 1982; Schwartz & Lacey, 1982). However, these observations still suggest no theoretical framework that might offer an explanation for the effects of both training paradigms on drug tolerance. The theory of Bolles (1972, 1975, 1979) on learning mechanisms and their occurrence in instrumental training paradigms has been especially helpful in this regard. So much so that during one of our discussions, I asked him if he had ever thought or intended his analysis of learning processes to extend to drug effects. His good-natured, enthusiastic disclaimer made it clear that such a theoretical excursion would remain my responsibility, although he might be willing to meet me if I arrived. We will begin the trip by describing Bolles's analysis of the learning process.

## Expectancy

Bolles has been one of the most influential theorists in the movement toward a more cognitive theory of learning. He has argued that the hypothetical mechanistic bond between a stimulus and response should be replaced by the associative concept, *expectancy*. This term derives from his view of learning as the acquisition of information about predictable relationships between events. The storage and retention of the information is an expectancy. The particular information that is acquired, of course, depends upon what events are associated. Each set of associated events provides different information and thus leads to a different type of expectancy. Bolles proposed that a Pavlovian conditioning procedure allows a subject to acquire knowledge about the relationship between a specific environmental stimulus (S) and some important event (S*). He termed the acquisition of this information a *stimulus–outcome* expectancy. During instrumental training, a subject's response (R) can be reliably associated with some important stimulus event (S*). Bolles considered that this R-S* pairing permits the acquisition of another expectancy, based upon information concerning the relationship between the response and the environmental outcome. This second expectancy was termed a *response–outcome* expectancy.

The evidence suggesting that instrumental training also can simultaneously involve classical conditioning led Bolles to propose that instrumental training could involve the acquisition of a stimulus–outcome expectancy and a response–outcome expectancy. His argument that instrumental training involves the development of both expectancies can be illustrated by returning to our simple example of an animal trained to bar press for food in a Skinner box. The important event here is food (S*), and it is contingent upon a bar press response (R), so the training reliably pairs R-S* events and permits the acquisition of a response–outcome expectancy. However, the environmental stimuli (S) of the Skinner box also are associated with the occurrence of S*, and the repeated pairing of S-S* permits the acquisition of a stimulus–outcome expectancy. It seems, then, that instrumental training provides a richer learning experience than Pavlovian conditioning because instrumental training conveys information that allows the acquisition of two expectancies about the occurrence of an important event: one based upon the stimulus environment and another upon a response.

From Bolles's perspective, expectancy is what is learned in *any* training situation. Whenever a stimulus or a behavior is repeatedly correlated with some important environmental event, an expectancy is acquired. The perception, encoding and retention of the information about such a relationship *is* the expectancy. The concept of expectancy is a hypothetical construct, related by specific rules to observable stimulus and response events. In this sense, it does not differ from a hypothetical *bond* that more mechanistic theories assumed tied stimulus and response events together. But the expectancy concept seems better able to predict and explain much of the variability that characterizes the display of a learned behavior.

In Bolles's theory, the occurrence of a learned response under instrumental training depends upon two considerations: A subject must have information that allows the acquisition of a response–outcome expectancy, and the expected outcome must have some desirable incentive value. With the expectation of a more favorable outcome, the probability of displaying the response increases. The theory implies that when a subject has acquired a response–outcome expectancy, a subsequent change in the value of the expected outcome should alter the occurrence of the response. For example, if the outcome is devalued, the occurrence of the response should be adversely affected. Support for this prediction and related hypotheses is accumulating (Colwill & Rescorla, 1986; Rescorla, 1987, 1990a, 1990b; Rescorla & Colwill, 1989).

Bolles's advocacy of a cognitive view of learning has been accompanied by an increased interest in cognitive processes in other areas of psychology. The term expectancy is now widely used as an explanatory concept. Although the usage of the term expectancy in other theories tends to vary, a review has identified some commonalities that are also consistent with Bolles's concept of expectancy:

> The term *expectancy* refers to an intervening variable of a cognitive nature. Whether explicit or implied, this cognitive variable is understood to be knowledge (information, encodings, schema, scripts, and so on) about relationships between events or objects in the real world. The term expectancy, rather than attitude or belief, is usually invoked when the author refers to the anticipation of a systematic relationship between events or objects in some upcoming situation. The relationship is understood to be of an if–then variety; *if* a certain event or object is registered *then* a certain event is expected to follow (although the *if* condition may be correlated with, rather than causal of, the *then* event). (Goldman, Brown, & Christiansen, 1987, p. 183)

One important feature of Bolles's learning theory is that it offers a means of testing causal relationships between behavior and the acquisition and content of expectancies. Much research in social and clinical psychology uses an expectancy concept similar to Bolles's in investigating the correlation between subjects' reports of expectancies and their behavior. But the causal relationship cannot be directly tested in such research. Goldman et al. (1987) have reviewed an impressive array of findings on alcohol use and abuse that may be attributed to learned expectancies. However, they too have stressed that a validation of the expectancy construct remains to be demonstrated, and will require experiments that manipulate the content of alcohol-related expectancies to demonstrate a causal effect on behavior. Our analysis of learned tolerance builds directly on Bolles's theory and aims to provide testable predictions about the influence of learned expectancies on behavioral tolerance to alcohol. Thus it may provide some needed evidence on the causal effects of expectancies. The possible contribution and relationship of our findings to theories concerning expectancies about drinking will be considered in Chapter 10.

# Theory

Bolles's analysis of the learning process in terms of expectancies provides a great step forward in our formulation of a theory of learned drug tolerance. His theory provides a basis for assuming that the learning occurring under Pavlovian and instrumental training is the acquisition of information. The difference between the two training procedures resides only in the information that is being learned. Of course, Bolles's theory was not concerned with the added complication of a drug. Thus his analysis of instrumental training dealt with a single important outcome, such as food (S*), and this same outcome was associated with the stimulus environment (S-S*) and with the response (R-S*). Training under a drug must consider this additional important drug stimulus (Sd*), but Bolles's theory seems otherwise applicable to such a situation. Thus tolerance developing under Pavlovian conditioning would presumably permit the acquisition of a stimulus–drug outcome (S-Sd*) expectancy. In contrast, tolerance developing during instrumental training allows the learning of both the S-Sd* expectancy *and* an expectancy concerning a response under drug and an environmental outcome (R-S*). The important feature of our analysis is that it suggests instrumental training under a drug can involve two *different* important outcomes. One is the drug stimulus (Sd*). The other is some important environmental event (S*). The information conveyed by a stimulus–outcome expectancy (S-Sd*) concerns the occurrence of the drug stimulus (Sd*), whereas the knowledge entailed in a response–outcome expectancy (R-S*) concerns the environmental consequence (S*). In other words, extrapolating Bolles's theory to instrumental training under drug involves the introduction of two important stimulus events. We still see that a stimulus and a response–outcome expectancy may be acquired, but the two expectancies differ not only on whether an environmental cue or a response predicts an outcome, but also on the sort of outcome that is expected. The total contents of the two expectancies now involve entirely different events. Speaking loosely, an individual expects that a certain situation, such as a reception, predicts the drinking of alcohol, and a certain response, like slurred speech, predicts a particular consequence (i.e., social censure).

When a subject receives alcohol and then performs a task, we now can identify the four events that provide the basis for two expectancies: (1) the environmental stimulus cues that precede the administration of the drug (S); (2) the drug stimuli (Sd*); (3) a behavioral response under the drug (R); and (4) its environmental outcome (S*). These events occur in a temporal sequence, and the general model is illustrated in Figure 3A. A reliable association between the first pair of events provides the opportunity to acquire a stimulus–outcome expectancy. A reliable relationship between the last pair of events permits the learning of a response–outcome expectancy. At present, our theory of learned tolerance is solely concerned with these two expectations. However, the figure shows that there also could be a temporal relationship between the drug stimulus (Sd*) and a response (R) that may provide an opportunity to acquire an additional intervening expectancy. If drug stimuli were reliably associated with a *particular* response, the acquisition of this information would allow a subject to expect to display a specific behavioral response after a drug is received. We will return to this idea in Chapter 9 where we consider responses to placebo drinks. For the present, we will confine our attention to some other interesting features of the two expectancies.

Figure 3A is a general model in that it represents the class of events involved in each expectancy. Experiments select and test instances of each type of event. Thus a Pavlovian conditioning experiment manipulates the relationship between some neutral environmental event (S) and the administration of a drug (Sd*) that evokes some particular response (R). This training situation involves an S-Sd* association. An R is also present, but its consequence (S*) is missing. The absence of any R-S* association during Pavlovian conditioning trials indicates that the training conveys no information that would allow the learning of a response–outcome expectancy. Thus our model here is consistent with traditional interpretations of

**A. THE GENERAL MODEL**

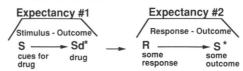

**B. THE MODEL FOR TOLERANCE**

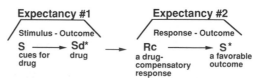

**FIGURE 3.** Task practice under a drug permits the acquisition of two expectancies. (A) The general model. (B) The model for tolerance.

the tolerance obtained in Pavlovian conditioning experiments. The entire effect is attributed to a learned S-Sd* association, stimulus expectancy for drug. But our model suggests that evidence on tolerance obtained in Pavlovian conditioning experiments may not tell the whole story. Their evidence is limited to stimulus expectancies for drug and cannot tell us anything about the effect of learned response–outcome expectancies on tolerance.

Experiments using instrumental training procedures to investigate behavioral effects of drugs likely include instances of each type of event shown in Figure 3A. Thus some particular environmental events (S) will be associated with the administration of a drug (Sd*), and some consequence (S*) will occur for a particular response (R) under the drug. The R-S* association in Figure 3A represents a generic response-outcome expectancy that stands for the combination of any one of many responses and consequences. For any given activity, the R may be drug-like or drug-opposite. Drug-like responses would be identified as symptoms of alcohol intoxication; drug-opposite responses would be recognized as symptoms of alcohol tolerance. Similarly, the S* may be any important event that confers advantageous or adverse consequences.

The response–outcome that may be learned depends upon the specific consequence of a particular response. For example, an experimenter may be interested in determining how one response (e.g, impaired bead stringing) is changed by the expectation of different consequences (e.g., money or electric shock). In this case, the R in our general model is specified and fixed, whereas the associated S* event is varied. This example is analogous to the conditions needed to test our hypothesis that alcohol tolerance is enhanced when a favorable consequence is associated with a drug-compensatory response.

Our interest in drug tolerance specifies that the particular response to be investigated is compensatory in character, opposite in direction to the behavioral effect of alcohol. We will designate a compensatory response as Rc. The association of some outcome (S*) with Rc permits the learning of a compensatory response–outcome expectancy. According to our hypothesis, a reliable association between Rc and a favorable outcome (S*) should enhance tolerance by increasing the occurrence of Rc.

Figure 3B presents the hypothesis schematically. It predicts that when stimulus expectancy for alcohol is present, tolerance is enhanced by the reliable association of a favorable S* with Rc. This model of learned tolerance involves the occurrence of two different important outcomes. One is the drug stimulus (Sd*) that is present in

Pavlovian training. The other is an environmental consequence (S*). Each may be important to a subject, but their values need not be correlated. The drug stimuli may be considered pleasant or noxious, quite independently of whether the outcome of a drug-compensatory response is pleasant or noxious. Figure 3B also shows that the events involved in each expectancy are entirely different, so it is possible to manipulate the events determining one association without changing the events involved in the other. This is an extremely important point because it means that the effect of different response-outcome expectancies can be investigated without altering the stimulus expectancy. We can change Rc-S* relationships by manipulating the S*. The S-Sd* events that govern stimulus expectancy for drug can remain unchanged. The independent manipulation of the Rc-S* expectancy is critically important because a convincing demonstration of its influence on tolerance logically requires that stimulus expectancy for drug is controlled. Thus, when stimulus expectancy for drug is held constant, the probability of observing tolerance should depend upon the Rc-S* association. A more valuable S* should increase the probability of observing Rc and enhance the display of tolerance. On the other hand, if S* is aversive, Rc may not recur, and drug effects may remain constant or intensify.

The model of learned behavioral tolerance, schematized in Figure 3B, also predicts the conditions under which task practice under alcohol will increase tolerance: Task practice should enhance tolerance if the display of drug-compensatory performance is reliably associated with some favorable environmental consequence. Under these conditions, task practice conveys information about this relationship that leads to the expectation of a desirable consequence for compensating for the effect of alcohol.

## Summary and Preview

This chapter has proposed a model of learned tolerance that assumes that learning consists of the acquisition of information about the relationship between events. A situation in which alcohol is received and some task is performed was analyzed for possible sources of learning. Two different pairs of events that could permit the learning of two different kinds of relationships were identified. One, symbolized by S-Sd*, involved the environmental stimulus context in which a drug was presented, and was considered to provide the information needed to acquire a stimulus expectancy for a drug. A second pair of related events concerned the response and its outcome, symbolized as R-S*. It was proposed that tolerance would be enhanced by the learning of a particular response–outcome relationship. This was the association between a drug-compensatory response and a favorable consequence, symbolized by Rc-S*.

This analysis of learned tolerance permitted a considerable refinement of our initial general question concerning the possibility that tolerance is affected by events after a drug is received. The analysis provided a specific hypothesis: Given that subjects expect and receive alcohol, the degree of tolerance observed should depend upon the desirability of the expected outcome of drug-compensatory performance.

The next step requires the development of an adequate experimental design to test the hypothesis with respect to social drinkers. We have seen that the use of a before–after design to investigate tolerance resulting from task practice under alcohol could not control stimulus expectancy for drug or exclude the possible effects of drug state dependent learning and functional demand. Our experiments will require a design that controls these factors and only treats groups differently with respect to the environmental outcome of performance under alcohol. Groups of subjects can be repeatedly presented with the same cues for drug administration, even though the consequence of drugged performance can differ for each group. By administering repeated doses to all groups under identical environmental conditions, the opportunity to acquire a stimulus expectancy for alcohol can be equalized among groups. Drug state and functional demand also can be controlled by requiring all groups to perform the same task equally often under drug. Thus this sort of experiment can control other factors that may affect tolerance, and test the separate effect of altering the consequence of drug-compensatory performance.

The next three chapters describe studies using this experimental design to investigate the alcohol tolerance of social drinkers. Because investigations of their alcohol tolerance are rare and the design is unique, Chapter 5 explains the methodological details of the studies.

# IV

ALCOHOL
TOLERANCE
IN SOCIAL
DRINKERS

# 5

## Research Strategy: Planning the Attack

**W**e have come a long way on the trail of puzzling instances of behavioral tolerance. The path first narrowed to events during performance under alcohol, and then to a particular class of R and S events. A jog in the direction of learning theory brought us to a model that specified how these events could combine to allow the learning of two expectancies. One pertained to the administration of a drug. This stimulus–outcome expectancy is represented as S-Sd*. A second expectancy concerned the consequence of behavior under the drug. This response–outcome expectancy, represented generally as R-S*, was considered to involve a drug-like (Rd) and a drug-compensatory (Rc) response. The theoretical model also identified one response–outcome expectancy, represented by the Rc-S* association, with our hypothesis that tolerance is enhanced by the expectation of a desirable consequence for a drug compensatory response. The model also implied the experimental design required to provide a decisive test of the hypothesis. The experimental design, methods, and procedures are explained in this chapter. The measures of the behavioral effect of alcohol that are used to infer tolerance are also described, as well as the operational definition of Rc and the Rc-S* relationships that determine the experimental treatments.

## Experimental Design

In order to design an experiment, we must be able to identify two pairs of empirical events that represent the S-Sd* and Rc-S* associ-

59

ations in our theory. The process of translating from theoretical to empirical events also helps to identify the important factors that must be controlled to test the effect of learned Rc-S* associations on alcohol tolerance. A concrete example perhaps makes the point most clearly.

Let us consider the experiment by Chen (1968) that was mentioned in Chapter 2 when before–after design studies were discussed. Chen tested the alcohol tolerance of rats that performed a temporal food maze. After the baseline training was completed, a behavioral group performed the task under repeated doses of alcohol. Another group performed the task before alcohol was administered, but was otherwise treated identically to the behavioral group. Our theory predicts that two associations, S-Sd* and Rc-S*, are each an important determinant of tolerance. Can they be identified in the treatment received by the behavioral group?

It is fairly easy to find S-Sd*. The repeated administration of alcohol (Sd*) was reliably associated with the environmental stimuli (S) that included the task. Thus the task apparently was a component in the stimulus events associated with the receipt of alcohol. The acquisition of a tolerance-enhancing S-Sd* expectancy in this situation may therefore include the task as a component of the cues leading the animal to expect alcohol. Now let us look for Rc-S*. The ataxic effect of alcohol would slow the animal's performance of a temporal maze so that it could not be completed within the time limit. However, compensating for the drug effect by running faster (Rc) would now be the response most reliably associated with the food reward (S*). Task practice under these conditions would seem to permit the acquisition of a tolerance-enhancing Rc-S* association. The animal may come to expect a desirable outcome of drug-compensatory performance. From our theoretical perspective, it appears that Chen's treatment of the behavioral group provided the opportunity to acquire both of the expectancies that favor the display of tolerance.

Now consider the treatment administered to the other group. Their task practice occurred without alcohol. A drug-compensatory response (Rc) would not be relevant to performance under these circumstances, and if a response does not occur, it cannot be associated with an environmental outcome (S*). This treatment therefore seems unlikely to have permitted the acquisition of any Rc-S* association. Now let us search for S-Sd*. The group had repeated administrations of alcohol (Sd*), but they were received after the animals had been removed from the task environment. It seems that the stimulus events (S) associated with Sd* specifically excluded the task. The animals may have come to expect alcohol in the presence of other environmental events, but the expectancy would be unlikely to include the task as a component in the S cues predicting alcohol. If anything, the control group may come to expect *no* alcohol in the presence of the task. When their task performance was subsequently tested under alcohol, the presence of the drug may have been quite a surprise. In sum, it seems that the treatment excluded *both* of the expectancies that could enhance tolerance.

Our review of the before–after design experiments in Chapter 2 mentioned that a Pavlovian conditioning analysis attributed the superior tolerance of the behavioral group to an S-Sd* association that permitted the animals to expect alcohol in the presence of the task. The inferior tolerance of the other group then was explained by the lack of opportunity to acquire this expectancy. Our analysis agrees with this interpretation, but goes further. From our perspective, an expectancy based upon S-Sd* is only half the story because it neglects the Rc-S* association. Thus our analysis would conclude that the behavioral group displayed greater tolerance because its treatment uniquely provided the opportunity to learn two expectancies; one concerning the occurrence of alcohol (S-Sd*) and another pertaining to the desirable outcome of drug-compensatory performance (Rc-S*).

This analysis pinpoints an important confounding that must be avoided in an experiment designed to test the effect of Rc-S* associations on alcohol tolerance. In experiments using a before–after design, one group has both of the tolerance-inducing expectancies, and the other has neither. When such groups are compared it is impossible to distinguish or separate the influence of the S-Sd* from the Rc-S* association, or to determine whether tolerance is affected by the Rc-S* association during task practice under alcohol.

Chapter 2 also mentioned that the tolerance displayed by a behavioral group in before–after design experiments has also been interpreted in terms of "functional demand." This hypothesis assumed that requiring the performance of some activity under a drug enhanced tolerance by increasing the ability of the drug to induce compensatory physiological adaptation. Our analysis offers another interpretation: Performing the task under alcohol provided the behavioral group with an opportunity to learn an Rc-S* association, whereas the drug-free task practice of the other group offered no chance to either display Rc or relate it to any environmental S*. In other words, task practice under alcohol is only likely to enhance tolerance when drug-compensatory performance is associated with a favorable consequence.

The analysis of experimental events that represent the variables in our theory identifies the important factors that have to be controlled in an experimental test of the effect of learned Rc-S* associations on alcohol tolerance:

1. All groups of subjects must have the same doses of alcohol. This ensures that the pharmacological exposure to the drug is equal in all groups.
2. All groups of subjects must have their doses of alcohol (Sd*) administered in an identical environmental context (S), so that all subjects have an equal opportunity to acquire the same stimulus expectancy for alcohol. This is an essential control because it equates groups on the tolerance-inducing effect of learning the S-Sd association in the experimental situation.
3. All groups of subjects must perform the task equally often under alcohol, so that the possible occurrence of a compensatory response (Rc) to alcohol is the same in all groups. This procedure also serves to equate groups for functional demand under the drug, and task practice under alcohol.
4. Each group of subjects receives a different outcome (S*) for the display of the drug-compensatory response. Thus the S* is the *only* factor that is manipulated in the experiment, and this changes the Rc-S* association that each group may learn.

This experimental design ensures that subjects of all groups are treated alike in all relevant respects except the S* associated with Rc. Under these experimental conditions, any group differences in behavioral tolerance to alcohol caused by changing the S* event in the Rc-S* association can be attributed to differences in the expected outcome of drug-compensatory performance.

There are many ways of manipulating S*. The effect of changing the incentive value of the S* associated with Rc is one example that could test our prediction that greater tolerance will be displayed by the group that expects a more desirable outcome for drug-compensatory performance. It is also possible to manipulate the opportunity to learn a given Rc-S* association. In this case, one favorable S* could be used, but the degree to which it is consistently associated with Rc would differ for each group. This would allow us to determine if a more reliable Rc-S* association results in faster learning, so that more tolerance is displayed sooner.

Experiments designed according to our list of requirements have been performed in our laboratory to collect evidence on these sorts of hypotheses. However, a description of the findings is best deferred until the procedure for conducting the studies is explained. These details are important because they allow investigators in other laboratories to repeat our experiments and check the evidence. The brevity of published articles does not permit a complete description of the procedures, and some variations, however slight they may seem, can actually change the entire experiment. An interesting example of this is provided in Chapter 7, where we discuss the development of our research on tolerance induced by mental rehearsal. An equally important reason for detailing the experimental procedure is that studies of social drinkers' tolerance to moderate doses of alcohol are uncommon, and the methodology is not well known. We will begin detailing our experimental procedure by describing the subjects and explaining the tasks they performed.

## Subjects, Selection, and Initial Briefing

Because of our interest in examining alcohol tolerance during the early stages of social drinking, our experiments selected subjects within the range of 19–25 years of age. All of the participants were men, and there were several reasons for using male subjects exclusively. One is that the information on their tolerance to alcohol is of special interest in view of statistics that show men in this age range to be disproportionately overrepresented in alcohol-related car crashes at low BACs (Simpson, 1975). The factors causing a high accident rate in these groups are unknown. It has often been suggested that young social drinkers may be *more* impaired than older social drinkers by a moderate dose of alcohol. But the reasons for their purported comparative lack of tolerance remain speculative. Thus research investigating factors that affect the behavioral tolerance of young male social drinkers may provide important practical information relevant to reducing their alcohol-related accident rate.

The use of male subjects also avoids some methodological difficulties posed by including women within the same experiment. An adequate comparison of the behavioral effect of alcohol in men and women requires that they be tested at the same BAC. However, the physiological differences between men and women, discussed in Chapter 1, indicate that their BACs can only be equated by administering a different, lower mg/kg dose of alcohol to women. They will attain a higher BAC if they receive the same mg/kg dose as men. There appears to be no convenient, reliable experimental procedure to adjust the alcohol dose of women to ensure that it yields rising and declining BACs equivalent to that of men. Recent evidence of a fetal alcohol syndrome in children born to alcoholic mothers also raises ethical concerns over the administration of any amount of alcohol to women who may be pregnant. This could occur inadvertently shortly after conception, before a woman may be aware she is pregnant. For purposes of an experiment, safeguards against this possibility are somewhat impractical. They would require pregnancy tests prior to each drinking session, or information concerning sexual activity and the use of contraceptives. Many women might find the collection of such information offensive.

The subjects in the studies were volunteers. The majority were university students who responded to notices posted throughout the campus requesting men aged 19–25 to participate in an alcohol study. Because subjects typically found the experiments interesting, they frequently recommended the experience to other students and to their friends in the community. As a result, we often had a waiting list of subjects for our experiments. The studies were approved by the Ethics Committee of the University Office of Human Research. Initially each volunteer was briefly interviewed to determine that he was in good health and had no history of any treatment for alcoholism or alcohol-related accidents. Individuals who reported taking no medication, and no problems involving alcohol, were considered to be potentially eligible. These persons were invited to a preliminary meeting to "find out more details about the requirements of the experiment before they decided to participate."

The briefing was conducted in a comfortable lounge in the laboratory. The potential participant was told that the experiment concerned the effect of moderate doses of alcohol on performance. The rather lengthy demands on a subject's time (six to seven appointments for a total of 14–16 hours) were explained, as well as the "honorarium" (about $3.00 per hour) for completing the entire experiment. The task that was to be performed and the equipment to measure BAC from breath samples were shown to the prospective subject. It was explained that complete details about a subject's drinks, BACs, and performance could only be provided when the experiment had concluded. The candidate for the study was also told that he must agree to abstain from all drugs for 24 hours, and to fast for 3.5 hours prior to a drinking session. The importance of having a standardized, light meal preceding the fast was also stressed. To ensure compliance with this rule, a menu was provided listing nonfat foods (e.g., clear tea, boiled egg, consommé) that could be consumed before beginning the fast, and other foods to be avoided (e.g., butter, cheese, french fries). A sample menu is shown in Appendix A.

Each individual was urged to carefully consider whether the time demands, fasting, and dietary constraints would pose any problem.

He was advised to agree to participate only if he felt he could fulfill the requirements, because they were absolutely essential for the experiment. When the requirements for participation were agreed to, the subject signed a consent form and completed a Drinking History Questionnaire (Vogel-Sprott, 1983). The questionnaire provided four measures of his alcohol use: dose (ml alcohol per kg body weight) that he usually drank on a social occasion; weekly frequency of such occasions; their typical duration; and an additional measure of "drink rate," obtained by dividing his dose by the duration of the occasion. The questionnaire and its scoring procedure are included in Appendix B.

The questionnaire measures were routinely used to compare the drinking habits of groups of subjects in an experiment. This may be a needless precaution in our studies because subjects' drinking scores have not correlated significantly with either impairment under the initial dose of alcohol or tolerance after repeated doses (Beirness & Vogel-Sprott, 1984b). The mean drinking habit scores of subjects in some of our experiments are shown in Appendix B.

One of the measures, dose per occasion, provided an additional screen for drinking problems. Age norms on dose per occasion reported by individuals in a national sample have been found to be significantly lower than the doses reported by persons of the same age who are receiving treatment for alcoholism or are charged with impaired driving (Duncan & Vogel-Sprott, 1978; Vogel-Sprott, 1983). Thus the mean doses reported by the 19–25-year-olds in the national sample could be used to compare the dose reported by a volunteer to determine whether it was within the normal range, or higher. All of the subjects who agreed to participate in our studies reported dose scores within the normal range.

The meeting was concluded by scheduling a set of appointments at approximately the same time each day, separated by at least 2 but not more than 10 days. A 2-day separation of appointments insured that a subject would not have to drink alcohol on consecutive days. The 10-day maximum interval was a matter of convenience, to allow tests of a subject to be completed within a 2-month period. Our studies have obtained no evidence to suggest that the interval between appointments affects a subject's performance. Subjects received a card listing their scheduled meetings, and a reminder phone call prior to each appointment.

The preliminary briefing attempted to reduce the loss of subjects from a study by ensuring that the obligations of serving as a subject were understood and accepted at the outset of an experiment. Few individuals found the requirements a deterrent. On average, probably no more than 5% of prospective volunteers decided not to participate in our research, and this was usually because the experiment required so much of a subject's time. The briefing appeared to serve its intended purpose because subjects who agreed to begin an experiment seldom withdrew, except for unforeseen events, such as illness, that were beyond their control.

# Apparatus

Our studies used two types of psychomotor tasks to assess behavioral tolerance to alcohol: a tracometer and a pursuit rotor. Details on each piece of equipment are presented in Appendix C, and a general description is presented here.

## The Tracometer

This is a subject-paced tracking task in which a subject works at his own speed to hit a set number of discrete target lights. To contact a target, a subject moves a steering wheel that controls a pointer on the target display panel. Whenever the pointer is centered on one target, a new target appears in a different position. The task was designed and built by the National Research Council of Canada (Buck, Leonardo, & Hyde, 1981). It is a particularly interesting task because tracometer performance has been found to discriminate among novice, experienced, and professional drivers (Engel, Paskaruk, & Green, 1978). Our studies assessed tracometer performance by the total time required to hit 100 targets. Performance becomes swifter with practice, so a smaller trial time score indicates better performance. After preliminary training, subjects usually complete a tracometer test within 2–3 minutes.

## The Pursuit Rotor

This psychomotor task is often used to demonstrate learning effects in undergraduate research courses in psychology. It requires a subject to track a rotating target with a hand-held stylus. The duration of a trial and the revolutions per minute (rpm) of the target are determined by the experimenter. The measure of performance is the time during a trial that the stylus is in contact with the target. Larger time on target (TOT) scores indicate more efficient tracking. In our research, the target rotated at 30 rpm, and a test of performance was based upon the average TOT during two 50-second trials that were separated by a 30-second rest. The duration of a test on the pursuit rotor was 3 minutes and was comparable to the duration of a tracometer test.

Some similarities and differences between the two tasks will be important to bear in mind when the results of our studies are presented. The first concerns the interpretation of the measures from each task. Better performance on the pursuit rotor is shown by *larger* TOT scores. In contrast, tracometer performance is better when targets are hit more swiftly, and this results in *smaller* scores because a trial takes less time to complete. The two tasks also appear to tap different psychomotor skills, because prior training on one task does not hasten learning of the other (Rawana, 1984). However, there is one important similarity between the pursuit rotor and the tracometer. Performance of these tasks seems to provide little in the way of knowledge of results or feedback about the adequacy of performance on a test. After subjects have been trained on these tasks, they find it very difficult to judge the adequacy of their performance from one test to the next. The addition of a tone signaling target contact appears to assist this judgement somewhat, but subjects still report considerable uncertainty in estimating their scores.Thus both tasks allowed an experimenter to present or withhold information about the adequacy of performance. The variable of informative feedback is important in the research to be discussed in later chapters.

## Blood Alcohol Concentration

Measures of BAC were estimated from breath samples. An experiment customarily used one instrument to measure BAC, with another as a standby. Details on the BAC equipment are provided in Appendix D.

# Experimental Procedures

Subjects were randomly allocated to different treatment groups when their appointments were scheduled during the introductory briefing session. Despite their group assignment, the treatment of all subjects was identical with respect to familiarity with an experimental task, drug exposures, stimulus expectancy, and task practice under alcohol. The procedures designed to control the influence of such factors are basic to all our experiments and will be described first.

## Familiarity with the Task Prior to Alcohol Administration

The tasks used in our studies had not been performed by subjects prior to entering an experiment. The use of an unfamiliar task in a study allows an experimenter to control individual differences in prior performance of a task. This is preferable to using something familiar, like typing or car driving, where subjects could begin an experiment with different degrees of prior skill. However, the use of a novel task also means that alcohol effects cannot be adequately evaluated without considerable prior drug-free practice. Otherwise, subjects would be learning the task while alcohol is also affecting their performance. The improvement in task performance because of learning might be canceled by the impairing effect of alcohol. The net effect could reveal no change in performance, and this may lead to the misleading conclusion that alcohol does not affect the performance of the task.

To avoid confounding the effect of alcohol with the initial learning of a task, subjects in our studies received considerable drug-free practice (24–30 practice tests) before alcohol sessions commenced. A subject's first two appointments were devoted to this training, and each practice session lasted approximately 1 hour. Our analyses of performance on the final six to eight tests of the second training session typically showed no significant continuing improvement over trials, so the tasks were fairly well learned by the conclusion of training. Although performance could still be expected to improve somewhat over the ensuing weeks of the experiment, this improvement was typically quite slight, and performance during any given day remained fairly stable. As a result of this training, a subject's drug-free test score on subsequent days provided a baseline measure of achievement on a task that was minimally affected by learning. Appointments in which alcohol was administered began after the training sessions, and a subject's score on his baseline drug-free tests preceding alcohol each day provided the criterion for assessing the alcohol-induced change in his performance during the drinking session.

## Exposures to Alcohol

The same dose of alcohol was administered to every subject during each drinking session in an experiment. The alcohol doses used in experiments were within the range of 0.62–0.66 g alcohol per kg body weight. This is a moderate dose, roughly equivalent to three or four 341-ml bottles of 5% beer for an average (70 kg) man. The beverage was administered in the form of three equal sized drinks, served at 20-minute intervals, and consumed within 5 minutes. In some studies, the alcohol was presented in the form of a cocktail containing 94.6% alcohol mixed with twice the volume of a carbonated soft drink that contained no caffeine. Because dealcoholized beer is a very credible placebo, some studies that used this placebo administered alcoholic drinks in 5% beer, fortified with 94.6% alcohol to reduce the fluid volume of beer needed for the dose. This resulted in smaller drinks that could be consumed within the time limits.

A subject's BAC was measured at 20-minute intervals. During the first 40 minutes, while the drinks were being consumed, any alcohol lingering in the mouth could influence a breath sample. For this reason, while drinking was underway the BAC was measured after subjects had rinsed their mouths with water twice. Rinses occurred when a drink was finished, and just before the breath sample that preceded the next drink. Under this dosing regimen, a rising BAC of about 50 mg/100 ml was usually obtained just before the third drink, 40 minutes after the session started. The typical curve of BAC resulting from the dose regimen is shown in Figure 4. A peak BAC around 80 mg/100 ml was typically observed by 60 minutes, and by 140 minutes the declining BAC was about 60 mg/100 ml.

The measures of BAC were obtained at the same intervals of every session of an experiment. This permitted the BAC measures to be analyzed to determine that the BACs of groups in a study were comparable, and that similar BACs occurred each time the dose was

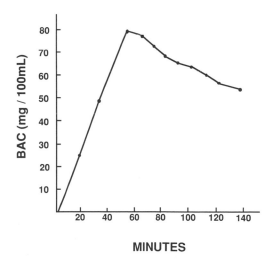

**FIGURE 4.** Typical blood alcohol concentrations resulting from the dose regimen.

repeated. These analyses have shown no significant differences in the BACs during sessions or among groups of subjects.

## Stimulus Expectancy

To ensure that all subjects had identical experience with the cues predicting alcohol, every subject in an experiment received and consumed his drink in a waiting room next to the task testing laboratory. The same types of glasses were used to serve all drinks, and the same person acted as the "bartender." Thus, within the context of an experiment, the set of environmental events (S) reliably associated with the receipt of alcohol (Sd*) was identical for every subject. With the same opportunity to learn the S-Sd* association, the tolerance-inducing effect of the expectation of alcohol should be similar for the subjects of all groups.

## Task Practice and Functional Demand under Alcohol

At regular intervals during an alcohol session, a subject left the waiting room and reentered the laboratory to perform a test on the task and provide a breath sample. Because each subject performed the same number of tests under alcohol, the possible effects of practicing the task, the sheer demand to function, and the probable occurrence of a compensatory response were comparable in all groups of subjects.

This description of the experimental control procedures provides the background information needed to understand how the behavioral effect of alcohol is measured and used to infer the occurrence of tolerance in our experiments.

# Behavioral Effect of Alcohol

When a subject arrives for a drinking session appointment, he first performs a few drug-free trials on the psychomotor task. The average of these scores provides a baseline criterion measure of his level of achievement that day. The effect of alcohol on task performance is measured by the difference between each of the subject's test scores under alcohol and his drug-free baseline score. The scores are subtracted to assess the alcohol-induced change in performance. Figure 5 illustrates the measures of change in a subject's performance during an initial session under the dose of alcohol. Here the zero

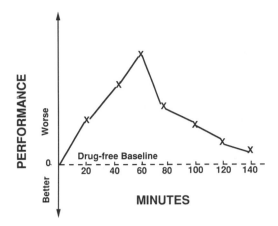

**FIGURE 5.** Alcohol effects on tests of performance during a drinking session. The average effect of the dose is the mean of the test measures.

point on the vertical axis represents the subject's drug-free baseline score prior to drinking. The degree to which test scores under alcohol differ from the subject's baseline indicates the drug effect. In the illustration, and in other figures presenting the results obtained with our psychomotor tasks, changes *above* baseline show *impairment*. In Figure 5, the degree of change in scores on successive tests during the session show impairment intensifying until the 60-minute period, where peak BACs occur. Thereafter, the impairment begins to diminish somewhat more rapidly than the BAC (cf. Figure 4).

A subject who is more impaired by alcohol during a test will show a larger change in his score. A change score is obtained from each of the regularly scheduled tests occurring during the rising and declining BAC of a drinking session. Figure 5 illustrates that the amount of impairment depends upon the particular BAC when the test occurred. Thus to obtain a more representative and reliable measure of the effect of a dose, our experiments measured the mean impairment obtained on all the tests administered during rising and declining BACs on a drinking session. The measure therefore represents the overall average effect of a dose and shows the degree to which a dose changes a subject's performance. The measure of the average effect of a dose provides the dependent measure for the evaluation of tolerance to repeated doses. If tolerance to a dose of alcohol develops as drinking sessions are repeated, then the average effect of the dose should become smaller on subsequent drinking sessions.

The behavioral data from the experiments are amenable to a number of different types of analyses. An analysis of variance of the average effect of the dose on drinking sessions has customarily been performed. Some studies have used the measures to calculate the rate of reduction in impairment on successive drinking sessions, and assess the resulting slope (i.e., rate of change in alcohol effects per session). Our studies have usually measured the average effect of a dose by the difference between a subject's test scores under alcohol and drug-free. However, another procedure that serves the same purpose is to analyze the test scores under alcohol, using a subject's drug-free performance score on the session as a covariate. When the data of an experiment have been assessed by this covariance analysis and compared with the analysis of measures of the change in scores under alcohol, the results have led to similar conclusions. There seems to be no reason to prefer one analysis over another. However, the covariance analysis results in statistically adjusted measures, whereas an analysis of the change in scores under alcohol provides untransformed measures that more directly reveal what was observed. Therefore, the effect of alcohol is usually presented in terms of the degree to which it changed performance from the drug-free level of achievement.

## Experimental Treatments

Equating groups with respect to so many factors that have been thought to induce tolerance may leave the reader wondering if there is anything left to manipulate and test. Indeed, ensuring that the exposure to these variables is equal for all subjects is unusual, but our studies are designed to examine a specific factor whose effect on tolerance has not previously been systematically investigated. This is the outcome ($S^*$) that is associated with a drug-compensatory response (Rc). Our experimental treatments present different Rc-$S^*$ associations to different groups of subjects. To provide this treatment, we use an operational definition to identify Rc and an Rc-$S^*$ relationship.

### The Definition of Rc

Learning studies usually train a response whose occurrence is directly observed. A bar press is one example. But our research concerns a drug-compensatory response, Rc, and it is not directly observable when a subject performs under a drug. How can we associate any environmental consequence (S*) with a response whose occurrence cannot actually be seen?

Our experiments provide a set of observations that permit an operational definition of Rc. First, the behavioral effect of an initial dose of alcohol can be readily demonstrated using our experimental tasks. Performance is initially quite reliably disrupted under a moderate dose of alcohol. When BAC is near a peak of 80 mg/100 ml, a subject's performance is usually only about 40% as good as his baseline drug-free level of achievement, and the measure of the average effect of the initial dose typically reveals about 12% impairment overall. Second, the observed effect of a drug is assumed to be the net result of a *constant* drug effect, plus a compensatory response to counteract the effect. Therefore, if a compensatory response increases, the drug effect must be seen to diminish. Finally, because our experiments measure the behavioral effect of alcohol on initial and subsequent drinking sessions, the initial and final effect of a dose can be compared to determine what change has occurred. The occurrence of tolerance is inferred when the behavioral effect of the final dose is weaker.

An extremely high degree of tolerance would be signified when a drug effect is no longer detectable. Such an observation would presumably indicate the occurrence of a very strong compensatory response. In our experiment, this could be detected by our measure of the change in a subject's performance under alcohol. The change would be zero because his test scores under alcohol and drug-free would not differ. Although such stringent evidence would not necessarily be required to infer the occurrence of a drug-compensatory response (Rc), this observation provides a good objective operational definition of Rc. Because the initial dose of alcohol reliably impairs a subject's task performance, he must be compensating for the drug effect when he displays nonimpaired performance that matches his drug-free achievement. Thus, in our research, the occurrence of Rc was operationally defined by a subject's test score under alcohol that equaled his drug-free test score.

## The Definition of an Rc-S* Relationship

The S* in our studies is some environmental event, such as a monetary reward, that is controlled by the experimenter. An Rc-S* relationship thus is identified by the degree to which the S* event is reliably associated with the occurrence of Rc, for example, a test score under alcohol that equals a subject's drug-free level of achievement.

This definition provides a basis for identifying different treatments that present different relationships between Rc and S*. Each group in an experiment is presented with a different Rc-S* association when they perform under repeated doses of alcohol. Thus the tolerance-inducing effect of the various treatments can be compared by measuring the subsequent effect of the alcohol dose in each group.


## Summary

This chapter has covered some rather unusual terrain. The description of how studies of alcohol tolerance in social drinkers can be conducted may be new to some readers. The development of an operational definition of a drug-compensatory response (Rc) in our research is a novel feature. The experimental design of the studies is also unusual because it plans to assess the tolerance-inducing effect of a treatment on subjects, even though they all also receive exposure to a host of other variables that may enhance tolerance. This is admittedly odd. It might even be considered risky. The exposure of all groups to so many variables that presumably induce tolerance could conceivably result in such a high and comparable degree of tolerance that no added effect of the experimental treatment could be demonstrated.

The actual risk is not so great. Although the subjects all receive the same exposure to many variables that may induce tolerance, clear evidence of their influence has so far only been provided for stimulus expectancy for drug (S-Sd*). Much research confirms that subjects will display more tolerance in the presence of stimulus cues that have been reliably associated with the administration of a drug. The provision of the S-Sd* association to all subjects in an experiment would permit them to learn to expect alcohol. Here we do run a risk of making everyone so alike in tolerance that the effect of our treatments may not be detectable. But this risk also offers a great potential gain. Suppose our treatments can be demonstrated to affect tolerance even while stimulus expectancy exerts its effect. This would provide much more compelling evidence for the importance of our Rc-S* treatment and would imply that two learned expectancies, S-Sd* and Rc-S*, affect tolerance.

# 6

## Alcohol Tolerance: Learning by Doing

Our theory suggested that the association between drug-compensatory performance and an environmental consequence could be learned when a task is perfomed under alcohol. This response–outcome relationship was designated as Rc-S*. The acquisition and retention of information about this association was termed an Rc-S* expectancy, and our analysis indicated that this expectancy should affect behavioral tolerance to alcohol.

The preceding chapter described the research strategy for an examination of this hypothesis. In order to test tolerance as a function of Rc-S*, experiments were designed to provide an operational definition of Rc, and to control other variables thought to induce tolerance. Our analysis proposed that alcohol tolerance depends, at least in part, upon a drug-compensatory response that has characteristics similar to instrumental responses in general. Therefore, by manipulating the association of S* with Rc, it should be possible to (1) enhance the acquisition of tolerance; (2) extinguish tolerance after it has been displayed; and (3) determine the degree to which behavioral tolerance on a task will transfer to a different task. The present chapter describes experiments testing these three hypotheses.

The test of tolerance acquisition is based upon the prediction that Rc is more likely to occur, and thus more tolerance should be observed, when a desirable S* is reliably associated with Rc. We will begin by describing research testing this hypothesis.

## Acquisition

Our research tested the effect of four different instrumental training procedures that commonly occur in everyday life. These conditions can be illustrated by an example that may strike a familiar chord. This concerns parental efforts to train children to do some new task, such as hanging up their clothes. If rewarding bribes are used, parents usually find that training is more effective with a bigger reward. They also quickly realize that it is often difficult to administer the reward consistently for a child's response and are dismayed to find that a reward is wasted if it occurs at various times not reliably associated with the new behavior. The inconsistent provision of a reward is as unlikely to train a new response as is a situation in which the response is not associated with any positive or negative consequence.

The preceding illustration depicts the effect of four different training procedures on the acquisition of a response. Two training treatments administer a large or a small reward contingent upon a response. The third administers a reward that is inconsistently associated with the response. The fourth treatment is essentially a null procedure in which the response has no environmental consequence. If these training treatments are applied to the Rc response, what happens to tolerance? The answer has been provided by some of our research (Beirness, 1983; Beirness & Vogel-Sprott, 1984a).

These studies involved four groups of subjects who performed the tracometer task. The experiments were designed according to our list of requirements described in Chapter 5. Thus the groups were equated with respect to other possible tolerance-inducing factors such as doses of alcohol, stimulus expectancy for drug, and task practice under alcohol. The groups were treated differently only *after* the dose was administered. The treatments manipulated *only* the outcome, S*, associated with the display of drug-compensatory performance, Rc. The operational definition of Rc was the attainment of a test score under alcohol that was as good as a subject's drug-free baseline score. Because an initial dose of alcohol impairs task performance, our definition of Rc assumes a subject must be compensating for the drug effect when he displays nonimpaired performance that matches his drug-free achievement.

A major purpose of the study was to test the hypothesis that tolerance is enhanced when a desirable S* event is reliably related to Rc. The reasoning here is that the opportunity to relate Rc to a favorable S* is offered each time the task is performed under alcohol. The accumulation of performance tests increases the reliability of the Rc-S* association. The expectancy concerning the desirable consequence of compensating for the drug effect should become more certain. Increasing the certainty of the expectation should enhance its influence: Rc should be more likely to recur, and so behavioral tolerance should become evident as the alcohol doses are repeated.

Two groups received training that provided a desirable S* contingent upon Rc. To test the hypothesis that the efficacy of such training is enhanced when the S* is more valuable, the value of the S* differed for each group. Subjects in one group (R) received a monetary S* (25 cents) for every test score under alcohol that was as good as their drug-free level of achievement. Subjects in the other group (I) received an informative S* that indicated the adequacy of performance on each alcohol test. This sort of information is some-times called "feedback" or "knowledge of results." It appears to be a desirable S* in its own right, because it has been shown to enhance the learning of a response (Schmidt, 1988). The 25-cent S* also conveyed informative feedback, but had the added attraction of financial gain. Thus the monetary S* was considered to be somewhat more valuable than the informative S*. Comparisons of the tolerance developed in the R and I groups tested the effect of the value of the S* associated with Rc.

The effects of the R and I training were also compared with two other control treatments that would be predicted to have little or no effect on tolerance. These two control groups performed the same number of tests under the doses of alcohol, but no S* was reliably associated with their Rc. To control for the possibility that just offering the money might affect behavior under alcohol, a random reward control group (RR) received 25-cent rewards equal to those earned by the R group, but the money was dispensed for alcohol tests selected beforehand, on a random basis independently of a subject's score on the task. Thus the 25-cent S* was not reliably associated with Rc. For this reason, the RR treatment would not be expected to have much effect on tolerance, even though money was administered for performance under alcohol. The other control group (N) received neither money nor information nor any other event contingent upon performance under alcohol. Because no S* was associated with Rc, N treatment was also predicted to have little effect on tolerance.

A different treatment was administered to each group during four drinking sessions. On each session, every group performed the task 12 times at regular intervals while BAC rose and declined. The alcohol-induced change in a subject's performance on the set of 12 tests measured the mean effect of the dose on each session. After subjects had completed their predrinking drug-free training on the tracometer, a test was usually completed within 120–180 seconds. The first dose of alcohol significantly slowed performance to a comparable degree in all groups. The mean effect of the first dose impaired performance on the tests and reduced overall efficiency by 11%. This meant that subjects took an average of 13–20 seconds longer to complete a test on the tracometer.

By the fourth drinking session, marked group differences were evident in the average effect of the dose. Figure 6 shows the mean effect of the fourth dose on each group. These data are presented in a fashion consistent with our earlier illustration of drug effects (see Figure 5). Thus the zero baseline in Figure 6 represents subjects' drug-free level of achievement just before drinking commenced. Scores above zero mean that alcohol slowed, and thus impaired, performance. A weaker effect of the dose is shown by smaller scores that are closer to the zero baseline. Scores below the baseline would mean that subjects' performance was better under the dose than drug-free. Because the groups displayed similar impairment under the first dose of alcohol, the differences now evident on the fourth dose demonstrate the occurrence of differential tolerance. The weakest drug effects, showing most tolerance, are displayed by the two groups, R and I, that had a valuable S* reliably associated with Rc. The R group had the 25-cent S*, and displayed somewhat more tolerance than the I group, whose S* provided information without any money. Significantly less tolerance was displayed by the other two groups, RR and N. Their impairment was fairly similar, even

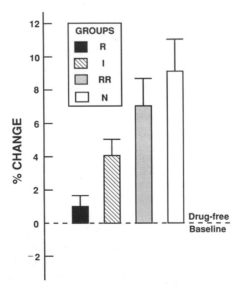

**FIGURE 6.** Mean effect of alcohol displayed by treatment groups during the fourth drinking session. A vertical bar shows the *SEM*.

though their treatments were very different. The RR group received the same number of 25 cent S* events as group R, but the occurrence of the S* was not reliably associated with Rc. In contrast, no S* event was administered for the performance of the N group. The one common component in the RR and N treatments was that no desirable S* was reliably related to Rc. Thus the evidence from the four groups is consistent with our prediction that the presence of a desirable Rc-S* association enhances the acquisition of tolerance to alcohol.

Our interpretation of the evidence in Figure 6 assumes that other tolerance-inducing variables cannot be acting to create the group differences we obtained. In fact, the experiment was specifically designed to ensure that subjects of all groups had the same exposure to these other variables. One of these, stimulus expectancy for alcohol (S-Sd*), could very likely be affecting the tolerance displayed by the groups in our experiment. However, all subjects had identical exposure to the S-Sd* sequence as well as such events as drug doses and task practice under alcohol. These effects thus may be assumed to be a constant component in the tolerance that all groups displayed. On logical grounds, these factors cannot explain, and would not predict, the group differences demonstrated in Figure 6.

Our interpretation of the evidence, of course, hinges upon the operational definition of Rc adopted in our experiment. We identified the display of a compensatory response (Rc) whenever performance under alcohol was equal to a subject's drug-free level of achievement. Because Rc cannot be directly observed when a subject performs under alcohol, our operational definition has the advantage of identifying Rc by empirical events that can be observed and confirmed by others. The definition is also compelling because it makes intuitive sense and appears to have face validity.

However, our conclusion that tolerance is affected by the expectation of a desirable S* consequence for Rc could be jeopardized if our operational definition is not a valid indicator of Rc. There is no way of directly verifying the occurrence of Rc under alcohol, because the behavioral response is an inevitable mix of the drug effect and Rc. However, support for an interpretation of treatment effects in terms of Rc-S* expectancies could be provided by demonstrating that the treatment will affect subsequent drug-free behavior in a predictable fashion.

## Demonstrating Rc-S* Expectancy Effects

Although Rc is not directly observable when a subject performs under alcohol, the disrupting effect of the drug provides good clues about the drug-opposite characteristics Rc should possess. Because alcohol slows tracometer performance, Rc should hasten reactions. If the Rc could be observed without alcohol, it should act to speed performance so that a tracometer test is completed more swiftly than normal. This facilitation would be detected by an improvement in performance that is superior to the drug-free level of achievement. Figure 6 helps to explain this idea. Here the change in performance above the drug-free baseline in each group showed impairment under alcohol. However, the degree of impairment differed among groups, and those who displayed smaller changes were more tolerant. We would attribute these differences to the training of different Rc-S* expectancies in each group. If this explanation is correct, then the change in performance displayed by each group in Figure 6 should be the reverse of what would be observed if alcohol were absent. For example, the weakest drug effect (i.e., most tolerance) was observed in group R, so this group should display the strongest Rc. This facilitating effect of Rc should be shown by a change in performance below the drug-free level of achievement. Least tolerance, indicated by the strongest drug effect, was shown in group N, so this group should display the weakest Rc.

Essentially, the prediction is that the four training treatments differently affected the occurrence of Rc. A test of this hypothesis requires a measure of Rc uncontaminated by alcohol. But an Rc is not relevant to a situation that clearly excludes alcohol: a drug-compensatory response would be unlikely to occur unless a drinker expected alcohol. To permit a measure of Rc in the absence of alcohol, our experiment included an additional drinking session that substituted placebo for alcoholic drinks.

The placebo session followed the fourth alcohol dose, whose effects on the treatment groups are shown in Figure 6. The events (S) associated with the administration of the dose (Sd*) on the preceding alcohol sessions had been identical for all subjects. Thus they had an equivalent opportunity to acquire the same expectation of alcohol. To ensure that subjects expected alcohol on the placebo session, the same cues predicting alcohol accompanied the administration of placebo drinks. From a subject's perspective, the placebo session was identical to all the prior alcohol sessions. The occurrence of Rc during placebo tests should result in faster, improved performance relative to the drug-free baseline, and would be shown by a change in performance below the drug-free baseline.

Other research has demonstrated that the expectation of a drug can enhance tolerance, so that a drug-compensatory reaction may be displayed when a placebo is received. Although this expectation may affect the results of our experiment, the subjects had been equated with respect to the opportunity to learn to expect alcohol. Thus the effect of this expectancy should be a constant component in the response to placebo that all groups displayed. In our study, stimulus expectancy for drug essentially provided a common background context in which all subjects would expect alcohol. The effect of stimulus expectancy could make the Rc of the four groups more alike. But it would not predict or explain group differences in the strength of Rc during the placebo session.

Figure 7 presents the mean change in performance under placebo displayed by the four groups when alcohol was expected. The changes below the drug-free baseline show each group improved performance under the placebo. This facilitation may be taken as a demonstration of Rc. It is not surprising to see some evidence of Rc in all groups, because they had a common background with respect to many factors that may induce tolerance and encourage a drug-compensatory response. A more important consideration here is that the treatment groups show differences in the strength of Rc *in spite of* their common background exposure to other tolerance-inducing factors. The contribution to Rc attributable to the background factors may be indicated by the results of the N group because it received our null treatment: No outcome of Rc was expected because Rc had no

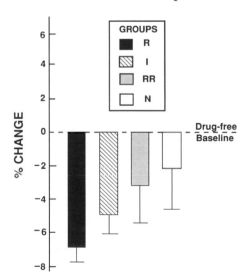

**FIGURE 7.** Mean response to a placebo when alcohol was expected. A vertical bar shows the *SEM*. Treatment groups had received four prior alcohol sessions. Their measures of tolerance to the fourth dose are shown in Figure 6.

associated S*. Figure 7 shows that the N group displayed the smallest compensatory reaction. The enhancement of Rc observed in the other groups should be due to their various Rc-S* expectancy treatments. The results from these three groups are in accord with our prediction. Groups R and I indicate that a stronger Rc occurs with the expectation of a more desirable S* for Rc. Group RR shows that when S* is desirable but only randomly related to Rc, the response is much weaker.

The placebo session demonstrated Rc uncontaminated by the effect of alcohol. The performance of the groups under the placebo (see Figure 7) is an exact reversal of their behavior under alcohol (see Figure 6). Thus the observations are consistent with the assumption that the group differences in alcohol tolerance were occasioned by treatments that altered the strength of a drug-compensatory response. The utility of our operational definition of Rc in the presence of alcohol is also indicated. The identification of the Rc and the S* event was required to create different Rc-S* associations. If our definition had not adequately identified Rc, our treatments could not have effectively manipulated Rc-S* associations. The adequacy of our operational definition of Rc is shown by the demonstration of treatment group differences in alcohol tolerance, and in the display of Rc when alcohol was expected.

The findings discussed in this section on acquisiton of tolerance have been detailed in other publications (Beirness, 1983; Beiness & Vogel-Sprott, 1984a). In sum, the evidence shows that alcohol tolerance is affected by events occurring after alcohol is received. This is an important point because the results cannot be explained by current theories of drug tolerance. Our theoretical analysis predicted the results and offered an interpretation that identified the cause with a learned relationship between two specific events, a compensatory response (Rc) and its outcome (S*).

However, there is another possible interpretation of the results that needs to be considered. It may have already occurred to the reader that the greatest display of Rc occurred in the group that was getting the largest reward for the response. Indeed, the tolerance and the response to placebo (see Figures 6 and 7) were observed while the groups were receiving their respective treatments. Thus it might be that the results simply demonstrate the incentive effect of a reward in enhancing the display of a response. Adherents of a traditional biological theory of tolerance would likely favor this idea. They might argue that the drug exposures allowed all groups to acquire a comparable Rc, and it was just more evident in the groups that had most to gain by displaying the response. In other words, the question is this: Is tolerance enhanced by learning to expect a desirable outcome, or is what we are seeing due to the value of the consequence at the time of test? The next set of studies was designed to address this question.

## Learning versus Performance of Tolerance

Although a training procedure may quite reliably improve performance, this change in behavior is often difficult to interpret. Performance may improve because of learning, or because of a willingness to display the response. The debate over learning versus performance effects of a training procedure has been a longstanding issue in the learning literature, extending back to the work of Tolman (1932), and the latent learning studies of Blodgett (1929). The same interpretation problem pertains to the treatment effects on alcohol tolerance that have just been described. This is because the effects were observed *while* different treatment conditions prevailed in each group. Thus it is possible that the R treatment induced most tolerance simply because it offered the greatest incentive to display this response.

Some of our studies of alcohol tolerance have attempted to determine the degree to which R treatment enhances the learning or the performance of the drug-compensatory response (Sdao-Jarvie, 1988; Sdao-Jarvie & Vogel-Sprott, 1991). This research was modeled on some studies that aimed to distinguish learning from performance effects of instrumental training treatments (e.g., Kimble, 1950; Smode, 1958). In these earlier studies, each group of subjects was initially trained with a different outcome (S*) for a response. The presence or absence of informative feedback, or winning points, are some examples of the S* used in these experiments. Of course, differences in the achievement displayed by the groups during the initial training period could be due to learning and/or to the incentive value of the S*. To assess the relative contribution of these two variables, a subsequent test administered the same S* for the response to all groups. If the groups' performance during the test did not differ, the evidence would imply that the different training treatments had resulted in a comparable degree of learning. Therefore, group differences in prior achievement could be attributed to the varied incentives (S*) used in the initial training. On the other hand, differences in learning during training would be indicated if group differences in achievement were maintained when groups were tested with the same incentive (S*) to perform. Studies in the instrumental learning literature have commonly found that a training procedure that leads to the best achievement is one that both enhances learning and provides a desirable incentive to perform (e.g., Smode, 1958).

The procedure of administering different initial training and subsequent tests under constant conditions was followed in our studies. These experiments also adhered to the list of design requirements described in Chapter 5 and were similar in several other respects to the research on tolerance acquisition that has just been discussed. The initial training phase of the study consisted of three alcohol sessions during which groups of subjects performed tests on the tracometer. During this period, each group received a different treatment that manipulated the S* associated with Rc. The next alcohol session was the test phase of the experiment. During this session, the same monetary-incentive (25 cents) S* was contingent upon the display of Rc by subjects of all groups. The results of this session thus tested the degree to which the tolerance displayed by the groups during their prior training treatments could be attributed to the learning of an Rc-S* association, or to the incentive effect of the S*. If the display of Rc had been determined by the incentive value of the S* during the prior treatments, then the alcohol tolerance of the groups should not differ on session 4. However, if the treatments had involved different learning opportunities, then group differences in tolerance should be maintained.

Our research with Sdao-Jarvie included a number of treatment groups. The results from four groups illustrate the findings on the learning versus performance effects of our treatments. Two of these groups received the tolerance-inducing treatments identical to those we have already explained and designated as I and R. Thus the Rc displayed by these groups was immediately associated with either an informative or a monetary (25-cent) S*, respectively. The other two groups received treatments that were predicted to have little effect on tolerance because no favorable S* was temporally contingent upon Rc. The N treatment (i.e., no S*), as described in the previous research, was administered to one of these groups. The other group (M) also earned 25 cents for displaying Rc on each trial, but the money was not dispensed until the conclusion of the experiment. Thus the S* was not temporally contingent upon Rc. Although the monetary incentive to display Rc in this group equaled that of the R group, the M treatment provided little opportunity to learn the Rc-S* relationship because no information about the occurrence of Rc in relationship to S* was provided.

The initial training phase commenced with the first drinking session. The impairment displayed by the treatment groups during this session did not differ significantly, but sizable group differences were evident by the third drinking session. The results during the third session were essentially similar to those described in the preceding section on tolerance acquisition. Thus most tolerance, that is, least impairment, was displayed by group R, that was receiving the 25-cent S* contingent upon Rc. Group I displayed slightly less tolerance. Least tolerance was displayed by the M and N groups, and the intensity of impairment displayed by these two groups did not differ significantly.

The learning versus performance effects of the treatments were tested on alcohol session 4. Before drinking commenced, all subjects were advised that 25 cents would be administered for the display of Rc on a trial under alcohol. Thus all subjects were informed in advance of the monetary incentive for displaying drug-compensatory performance. Prior training history was the only systematic factor differentiating the groups. The tolerance displayed by each group on session 4 is shown in Figure 8. Here again changes above the zero baseline indicate impairment, and less impairment means a weaker drug effect (i.e., more tolerance). The data show that greater tolerance continued to be displayed by the groups with a training history of R and I. Those that had M and N training displayed an abrupt increase in tolerance when the monetary S* was introduced on session 4. However, these groups were still significantly more impaired than groups R and I. The carry-over effects of training on this test session imply that the treatments involved learning, not simply incentive.

The enduring effect of training history was also confirmed in

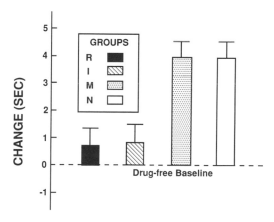

**FIGURE 8.** Mean response to alcohol by groups with different treatment histories. A vertical bar shows the *SEM.*

response to placebo when alcohol was expected. These results were obtained by administering a fifth drinking session to the groups. This session continued to dispense a 25-cent S* for Rc but substituted a placebo for alcohol. Figure 9 shows the response to placebo of the groups with different training histories. The change in performance below the drug-free baseline reveals improvement, a compensatory facilitation indicative of Rc. The influence of treatment history endured to affect the response to placebo. The groups with a history of R or I training continued to display the strongest compensatory reaction.

These findings provide a clear "yes" to the question, "Does learning to expect a desirable consequence for compensation *itself* enhance tolerance?" Our reply is affirmative because the differences in the tolerance observed under the initial training conditions remained evident on subsequent alcohol and placebo sessions that provided all groups with the same incentive to perform. Now how can this be explained? The R and I treatments were the only ones designed to provide information about the association between a compensatory response and a desirable consequence. The expectancy resulting from the acquisition and retention of this information should have enhanced the likelihood of immediately displaying compensation. In this sense, drinkers who have learned to expect a desirable consequence for compensating for alcohol have a "head start" on tolerance.

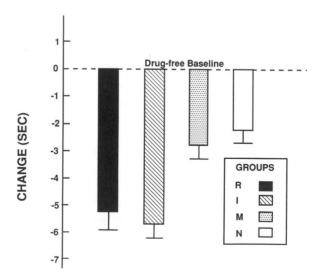

**FIGURE 9.** Mean response to placebo by groups with different treatment histories. A vertical bar shows the *SEM.*

The results also give a clear "no" to the suggestion that tolerance is governed *solely* by the value of the S* present when tolerance is tested. But this does not mean that the incentive value of S* has no effect. Our experiment did detect some tolerance-enhancing effect of presenting the 25-cent S* for Rc. This was suggested by the abrupt reduction in the alcohol-induced impairment displayed by the M and N groups when the monetary S* was introduced on the alcohol test session.

In sum, the findings lead to the conclusion that training a reliable association between Rc and a desirable S* had both learning and incentive effects that increased the display of tolerance. This conclusion is consistent with earlier instrumental learning studies of training effects. Our evidence is also in line with some animal research on drug tolerance that demonstrates a rat's prior drug-free behavioral history can affect its response to the first administration of a drug (Barrett, Glowa, & Nader, 1989). However, the evidence on training history has typically not addressed the question of what is being learned. It has also been noted that a major problem with most studies of instrumental learning effects on behavioral tolerance is their inability "to specify what, precisely, is learned when a subject compensates for the initial disruptive effect of the drug" (Wolgin, 1989, p. 88).

Our research differs from others in that it is designed to test the hypothesis that what is learned is information about the relationship between a particular set of events. The learned information that induces tolerance concerns the association between compensatory performance (Rc) and a desirable outcome (S*). When the information is learned, it is represented as an Rc-S* expectancy that increases the occurrence of Rc so enhanced tolerance is observed.

If our interpretation is correct, we should be able to do some sleight of hand tricks with alcohol tolerance. After the Rc-S* expectancy is trained and tolerance is displayed, we should be able to make tolerance disappear, or reappear in the performance of a different task, just by changing the S* event in the Rc-S* relationship. In the technical terminology of learning, these phenomena would be called *extinction* and *transfer of tolerance,* and tests of these hypotheses will be considered next.

## Extinction

Biological and pharmacological theories of tolerance assume that the action of a drug causes tolerance, and therefore the drug administration must stop if tolerance is to subside. In contrast, our theory predicts that behavioral tolerance to alcohol can be extinguished without stopping the administrations of alcohol. All that is needed is to withhold the desirable S* a subject has learned to expect for tolerance (Rc). Support for this hypothesis has been provided by research that administered R treatment to develop alcohol tolerance. Then, during additional alcohol sessions that withheld the desirable S* for Rc, the extinction of tolerance was demonstrated (Mann 1980; Mann & Vogel-Sprott, 1981).

A description of one of our studies (Mann & Vogel-Sprott, 1981) illustrates these findings. This experiment involved a total of six drinking sessions. The alcohol dose regimen was the same as our other studies, and all subjects received their drinks under identical environmental conditions. A pursuit rotor task was used to assess performance, and drinking sessions began after preliminary training on the task. The first four drinking sessions trained the group R subjects to expect a desirable consequence for compensating for the effect of alcohol. Thus group R performed the task under the drug five times during each session and received a 25-cent S* for the display of Rc. The Rc was again identified as a test score under alcohol that equaled the subject's drug-free level of achievement. The last two alcohol sessions tested extinction. They were conducted in an identical fashion except that the 25-cent S* was withheld, so Rc no longer had any environmental consequence.

The study also included two control groups. An N group provided a control for alcohol exposures and task practice under alcohol. The N group was treated exactly like R, but received no S* for performance and therefore had no opportunity to learn any Rc-S* association. The second group (P) provided a control for presenting the monetary S* on tests after drinking. The P group received placebo instead of alcoholic drinks, but was otherwise treated exactly like group R. Thus subjects in group P also performed the task five times after drinking on each session and received 25 cents for every test score that equaled their drug-free level of achievement. However, the P treatment provided no opportunity to learn the Rc-S* association because their drinks contained no alcohol and no compensation (Rc) for drug effects was involved. When extinction was tested during the last two drinking sessions, group P continued to receive a placebo, but the S* was withheld. Group N continued to receive alcohol with no S* event.

During the first drinking session, the dose of alcohol impaired the performance of groups R and N to a similar degree, about 16%. In contrast, the performance of the P group did not change significantly from their drug-free baseline achievement prior to drinking the placebo. The performance of the groups on the last drinking session before the extinction test sessions began is shown in Figure 10A. Changes above the baseline show impairment, and are negative because poorer scores on the pursuit rotor task are smaller. This means that the time on target during a test is less. The group mean scores show that the R group is most tolerant and only slightly impaired by the alcohol dose, whereas the N group is considerably more impaired. These results are essentially similar to those obtained with R and N treatments on the tracometer task. The effect of paying subjects to maintain their drug-free level of achievement after drinking a placebo is indicated in group P. Their performance is slightly but not significantly better than their drug-free level, and it is not significantly different from that of group R.

The mean change in performance displayed by each group during the two extinction sessions is presented in Figure 10B. The tolerance previously displayed by group R is no longer evident. With the withdrawal of their expected reward for drug-compensatory performance, the impairing effect of alcohol was again displayed. The extinction of tolerance in the R group cannot be attributed to a general loss of incentive to perform the task when a monetary S* was removed, because the performance of the placebo group, whose money also was withdrawn, showed little deterioration from baseline efficiency.

In sum, the extinction of behavioral tolerance to alcohol despite

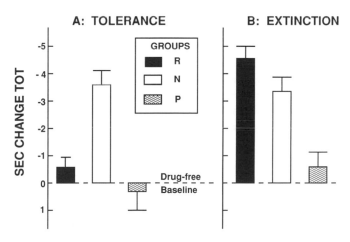

**FIGURE 10.** Training and extinction of tolerance. (A) Session 4 mean change in performance after drinking alcohol (groups R and N) or a placebo (group P). Groups R and P received money for compensatory performance. Group N had no money. (B) Session 5 mean change in performance when money was withheld from groups R and P. A vertical bar shows the *SEM*.

continued drinking is a very robust phenomenon. It cannot be explained by a physiological exposure interpretation of alcohol tolerance. Studies have shown that manipulating the S-Sd* expectancy can affect tolerance: Administering alcohol without the environmental cues that predicted the drug can reduce tolerance. But this cannot account for the evidence of our experiment because the S-Sd* expectancy based upon cues for alcohol was held constant. Other theories thus do not explain or predict the extinction of social drinkers' behavioral tolerance to alcohol demonstrated in our experiment; our theory does.

# Transfer

Our theory has led to evidence on the transfer of tolerance that also cannot be explained by existing theories. These findings are of considerable interest because others have attributed the transfer of tolerance to a homeostatic compensatory reaction induced by alcohol exposure (LeBlanc, Gibbins, & Kalant, 1975b). This conclusion was based upon research showing that animals that had developed tolerance to the effect of alcohol on the performance of one task also displayed tolerance when a different task was performed for the first time under alcohol. One task required solving a circular food maze within a time limit. The other required walking on a moving belt to avoid falling on an electrified grid. The tasks were different in that learning one did not influence the learning of the other. However, the tasks were similar in that compensating for the behavioral effect of alcohol was rewarded by the attainment of food in the maze, and avoidance of shock on the moving belt task. The provision of a desirable consequence for a drug-compensatory response on both tasks suggests that exposures to alcohol may not adequately account for the transfer of tolerance in the LeBlanc et al. (1975b) study.

The transfer of alcohol tolerance on one task to a different one may be affected by the presence or absence of the desirable S* a subject has learned to expect for the display of tolerance (Rc). Some of our experiments have tested this prediction (Rawana & Vogel-Sprott, 1985). In this research, drinkers received repeated doses of alcohol and performed a task (task 1) under alcohol when a monetary S* was contingent upon drug-compensatory performance (Rc). The training phase of the experiment concluded when tolerance was displayed. An additional drinking session examined transfer by testing performance on another task (task 2) under alcohol when the

S* was either present or absent. The two tasks used in the experiment were the pursuit rotor and the tracometer. They were analogous to the two tasks used by LeBlanc et al. (1975b), in that learning one does not affect the learning of the other (Rawana, 1984). Subjects received preliminary training on both tasks before alcohol sessions began. The dose regimen and presentation of alcohol during drinking sessions were identical for all subjects.

Task 1 was performed during the first four drinking sessions. One group, R, performed the task after drinking and received a 25-cent S* contingent upon drug-compensatory performance (Rc). The R treatment thus provided an opportunity to acquire an Rc-S* expectancy. Another group served as a control and received "rest" treatment, in which the task was performed *before* alcohol was received. Our "rest" treatment was analogous to the control condition used by Chen (1968, 1972) who administered task practice before alcohol. When the "rest" subjects received alcohol, their BACs were measured and they remained otherwise at leisure in the laboratory. Thus the "rest" group received the same doses of alcohol as group R. They also performed task 1 equally often and received the 25-cent S* for maintaining their drug-free baseline level of achievement. The important single different feature of the "rest" treatment was that task 1 was performed drug-free, just prior to drinking. Performance in the absence of alcohol should entail no drug-compensatory response, and thus the "rest" treatment presumably provided no opportunity to learn the Rc-S* association.

The fifth drinking session concluded the training phase of the experiment. This session tested the tolerance on task 1 that resulted from the R and "rest" treatments. To equate groups on the incentive to display Rc during this session, a 25-cent S* was administered to all subjects for drug-compensatory performance on tests under alcohol. The results are shown in Figure 11A. After four sessions of R or "rest" treatment, the R group displayed significantly more tolerance on task 1 than did the "rest" group. It is worth emphasizing that these effects were evident *even though* both groups were receiving the 25-cent S* for Rc during this tolerance test. The incentive to display tolerance was equivalent. Further, subjects with the history of R treatment performed task 1 slightly better under alcohol than they performed drug-free. The R group was displaying fairly complete tolerance to the dose because the effect of alcohol was essentially undetectable. In contrast, subjects with a history of "rest" treatment continued to display significant impairment on task 1.

The transfer of tolerance was tested on the sixth session, when all subjects performed task 2 for the first time under alcohol. To test the

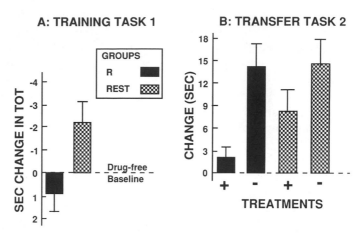

**FIGURE 11.** Training and transfer of tolerance. (A) Mean effect of alcohol on task 1 performance after groups had received R or "rest" treatment. (B) Transfer of tolerance to task 2 when half of the R and the "rest" groups received money ( + ) for compensating, and the remainder received no money ( − ). A vertical bar shows the *SEM*.

effect of the presence ( + ) or absence ( − ) of the S* on the transfer of tolerance, each treatment group was divided. Half the R group ( + ) received the same 25-cent S* they had learned to expect for compensatory performance on task 1. The S* was withheld for the performance of the other R subgroup ( − ), so the expected consequence for compensation was not confirmed when they performed task 2 under alcohol. It was also important to determine that differences between the two R subgroups during the transfer test were not simply due to the presence or absence of the S*. For this reason, half the "rest" group ( + ) received the 25-cent S* for drug-compensatory performance on task 2, and the remainder ( − ) had S* withheld.

Figure 11B shows the effect of treatment history on the transfer of tolerance to task 2 when the advantageous S* for Rc was present or absent. The R group had previously displayed tolerance when task 1 was performed. The transfer of their tolerance to task 2 was significantly affected by the presence ( + ) or absence ( − ) of the expected consequence of compensatory performance. Tolerance readily transferred and was very well retained *only* when the expected desirable consequence continued to occur. When the S* was absent, little transfer was evident. Considerable impairment was displayed on task 2 when the S* was absent, and the degree of impairment was similar whether subjects had a history of R or "rest" treatment. A comparison of the effects of the + and − conditions on the groups that had "rest" treatment showed that the addition of the S* for compensatory

performance on the transfer task reduced impairment. The Rc-S*
contingency provided to this latter group should have provided these
subjects with an opportunity to begin learning the Rc-S* association.
Such learning could explain why the "rest+" group with money
displayed less impairment on the transfer test than did its counter-
part, "rest − ", without money. Additional evidence supporting our
hypothesis is provided by comparing the "rest" and R groups under
the + condition. Both received S* for compensating on the transfer
task, but the R group was significantly more tolerant. The only
difference between these groups resided in their task 1 training
history. Group R had the opportunity to acquire the expectation of a
desirable outcome for compensatory performance prior to the test of
tolerance transfer. The "rest" group had no such learning opportunity. These results imply that an established Rc-S* expectancy itself
facilitates the transfer of tolerance to another task.

The results of our tolerance transfer research directly challenge
the conclusion (LeBlanc et al., 1975b) that the transfer of alcohol
tolerance between two motor tasks is a result of some neuronal or
central nervous system adaptation to the presence of the drug in the
body. That interpretation was based upon an experiment in which the
training and transfer tasks each provided a reliable reward for
drug-compensatory performance. This condition was represented in
our experiment by the R training and the + transfer test: the training
and the transfer task both provided a reliable reward (S*) for
compensating (Rc). The strong transfer of tolerance displayed under
this combination of conditions in our research is also consistent with
the evidence of LeBlanc et al. (1975b). However, our study included
additional groups to manipulate the consequences of drug-
compensatory performance. The occurrence of physiological adaptation to alcohol cannot account for the lack of transfer when S* was
absent. In contrast, the transfer of alcohol tolerance observed in this
research is predicted and explained by the expected consequences of
drug tolerance.

## Summary and Implications

This chapter described evidence demonstrating that behavioral tolerance to alcohol is affected by learning the association between a
desirable consequence (S*) and drug-compensatory performance (Rc)
under alcohol. The occurrence of Rc was identified by the elimination
of impairment under alcohol, so that a subject's performance re-

turned to his drug-free level of achievement. Experiments consistently demonstrated that changing the S* associated with Rc altered tolerance to alcohol, as well as the strength of a drug-compensatory reaction to a placebo when alcohol was expected. The reliable association between an advantageous S* and Rc enhanced tolerance, whereas the same S* randomly related to Rc had little effect. The experiments also indicated that the tolerance-enhancing effect of the Rc-S* association could be attributed to learning this response–outcome expectancy, and to the incentive value of S*. In addition, after subjects were trained to expect the Rc-S* association and tolerance was displayed, their tolerance could be extinguished by withholding the S*. This extinction was remarkable because it occurred even though drug administrations and the expectation of receiving alcohol continued. Moreover, the tolerance displayed in one task when the Rc-S* was expected also readily transferred to a different task, but *only* when the same S* was associated with Rc on the second task. This evidence on the transfer of alcohol tolerance, too, was unusual in that it could not be explained or predicted by theories of tolerance based upon the physiological effect of exposure to alcohol or of stimulus expectancy for the drug.

The results of the research in this chapter bear on the puzzle of what causes social drinkers to acquire a high degree of behavioral tolerance to alcohol. It has previously been attributed to repeated drug use, or learning to expect alcohol as doses are repeated, or task practice under the drug. However, these factors were all controlled in the experiments described in this chapter. Therefore, they cannot explain the pronounced variation in the behavioral tolerance demonstrated by social drinkers. The evidence clearly implies that an account of social drinkers' tolerance requires consideration of some additional factors. Our experiments identified one important causative factor: learned information about the Rc-S* relationship. Moreover, the effect on tolerance of manipulating the S* associated with Rc was strikingly similar to the effect obtained by manipulating the consequence of an instrumental response.

Instrumental behavior is characterized by cognitive and perceptual processes of a voluntary nature. Demonstrations that tolerance is predictably altered by manipulating the Rc-S* association suggests that the same characteristics may apply to social drinkers' behavioral tolerance to alcohol. Our interpretation of what is being learned that affects tolerance developed from Bolles's view (1972, 1975, 1979). Thus the learning is assumed to depend upon information about the relationship between Rc and S*, and the retention of this information provides an Rc-S* expectancy that affects alcohol tolerance. Such an interpretation implies that other means of acquiring information about the Rc-S* association should affect tolerance the same way as firsthand experience of the response and its environmental outcome. Thus it may be that tolerance can be acquired without overtly performing under alcohol. Mental rehearsal is one learning technique that involves no overt activity. Perhaps the repeated mental rehearsal of the Rc-S* association under alcohol may enhance behavioral tolerance to the drug? The next chapter reports experiments pursuing this hypothesis.

# 7

## *Alcohol Tolerance: Learning by Thinking*

**F**amous artists and writers have occasionally claimed that thinking under the effects of a drug inspired new behavior. But the notion that thoughts under alcohol may inspire behavioral tolerance seems farfetched indeed. Nonetheless, our analysis seemed to point in this direction.

In theory, information about the relationship between compensatory performance (Rc) and a desirable consequence (S*) enhanced alcohol tolerance. The repeated imagined association between the mental representation of Rc-S* events seems analogous to repetitions of overt Rc-S* events in the environment. If mental and overt practice involve the same information, then both modes of training should have similar effects on tolerance.

Mental practice is the "symbolic rehearsal of a physical activity in the absence of any gross movements" (Richardson, 1967a, p. 95). This training is also variously termed mental rehearsal, imaginary practice, introspective rehearsal, symbolic rehearsal and conceptualizing (Egstrom, 1964). Mental rehearsal has often been administered to train skill in sports and is generally believed to be extremely helpful. However, its practical application in the sports arena cannot provide the experimental evidence needed to evaluate the effect of mental rehearsal. Mixed results have been obtained in motor skill experiments comparing the effect of overt, mental, and no practice (i.e., rest). Some studies find mental rehearsal as valuable as overt practice in learning a motor task (e.g., Oxendine, 1969; Rawlings, Rawlings,

Chen, & Yilk, 1972). However, more recent research has led to a more conservative conclusion. Reviews of the literature (Druckman & Swets, 1988; Feltz & Landers, 1983) have concluded that mentally practicing a motor skill is only *somewhat* better than no practice at all. Although some evidence does show mental rehearsal facilitates motor learning, the "diffuse nature" of mental rehearsal makes it difficult to explain (Druckman & Swets, 1988). Various theories have attempted to account for mental rehearsal (e.g., Corbin, 1972; Gould, Weinberg, & Jackson, 1980; Richardson, 1967a, 1967b), but the phenomenon remains poorly understood.

In sum, the literature on mental rehearsal provided slim encouragement for its use in studies of alcohol tolerance. The essential conditions for the successful application of mental rehearsal training had not been identified, even for the comparatively simple case of psychomotor learning without any drug. Thus we were faced with a doubly discouraging task. Our theoretical hypothesis concerning alcohol tolerance induced by mental rehearsal seemed incredible, and there was no proven effective procedure for applying the mental training. Fortunately, serendipity took a hand at this stage and provided an encouraging clue.

In order to practice the experimental procedures, a new experimenter in our laboratory conducted a pilot study that included our "rest" treatment. This treatment administers repeated doses of alcohol to subjects who perform the task drug-free, before drinking alcohol. Chapter 6 described the "rest" treatment used in our tolerance transfer research, and showed it to have no tolerance-enhancing effect. This finding has been repeatedly confirmed since Chen (1968) first used this treatment. However, the "rest" treatment administered by the new experimenter of the pilot study resulted in an astonishing degree of tolerance. The mass of evidence demonstrating that "rest" treatment has no such effect on tolerance indicated that the pilot study must have altered some important feature of this treatment. However, the source of this effect was difficult to identify because no aspect of the experimental protocol appeared to have changed. The search was analogous to looking for the proverbial needle in a haystack.

A verbatim record of the comments between the subjects and the experimenter finally detected one minute variation that occurred after drinks were served. Under the "rest" treatment, subjects' BACs are regularly measured after the dose is received, but subjects are otherwise free to entertain themselves. While subjects were providing breath samples to determine their BACs, the experimenter occasionally asked subjects to think about doing the task and guess how well they might perform. Subjects usually thought for a few minutes and then made a guess as to whether their performance would be equal to their drug-free performance. This question–answer interchange was the unique innovation. The experimenter considered it natural to include the question because subjects would otherwise think it odd to do all their task practice before drinking. In addition, the experimenter reported that the question seemed to increase subjects' interest because they then often appeared to be thinking about performing the task when their BACs were measured.

Could it be that the introduction of this one casual question transformed our "rest" treatment under alcohol to one in which subjects were spontaneously mentally rehearsing the task? If a haphazard occurrence of mental rehearsal under alcohol caused the tolerance that had been observed, a systematic examination of mental rehearsal should be very fruitful! This chapter presents the fruits of the research. Findings are presented on the equivalence of mental and overt task practice effects on behavioral tolerance to alcohol, the interpretation of mental rehearsal effects, and the provocative prediction that mental rehearsal may induce tolerance *without* repeated doses of alcohol.

## The Equivalence of Mental and Physical Practice

Is alcohol tolerance enhanced by mentally rehearsing the association of drug-compensatory performance (Rc) with a desirable outcome (S*)? How do mental rehearsal (MR) effects compare with those obtained through performance that associates overt Rc and S* events? The MR experiments testing these sorts of questions were similar to our other studies in terms of subject selection, briefing, and preliminary training on a task. Drinking sessions were also scheduled at approximately weekly intervals. In addition, the dose regimen, measure of alcohol-induced change in performance, and the criteria of compensatory performance (Rc) and tolerance were identical.

Mental rehearsal treatment consisted of the administration of a dose of alcohol followed by a set of mental rehearsal trials. Each trial was guided by taped instructions to ensure that the duration was equivalent to the duration of a test of overt performance. The recorded message asked subjects to imagine specific movements involved in the task, and to assess the adequacy of their performance on each imaginary trial. An example is given in Appendix E by a transcription of the tape used to guide mental rehearsal of the pursuit rotor task.

The MR treatment required one change in our customary experimental procedure. Because no overt performance occurred during mental rehearsal, its effect could only be assessed by adding a pre- and a posttreatment session that measured the behavioral effect of the alcohol dose. This meant that all the other groups in an experiment also had to receive the pre- and posttreatment assessment, and it had to be conducted under identical conditions for all groups. In our research, the pre- and posttreatment sessions measured alcohol effects when all groups performed a task with a monetary outcome (S*) for compensatory performance (Rc). This is the R treatment that was described in Chapter 6. Its use during the pretreatment session seemed to be a prerequisite for the group that was to mentally rehearse, because the tasks in the studies were ones that subjects had never performed under alcohol, and such an experience was likely needed to enable subjects to imagine drug-compensatory performance and its outcome. In order to equate the groups, the R condition had to be used in the pretreatment sessions of all groups. This had the disadvantage of providing all subjects with an initial experience that could foster a tolerance-enhancing Rc-S*. Thus the pretreatment session created a risk of making groups more alike, so that MR effects on tolerance would be more difficult to distinguish.

The determination of the treatment-induced change in the effect of alcohol had to be based upon pre- and posttreatment measures obtained under identical conditions. Therefore, the posttreatment effects were also assessed under the R condition. This again provided more training of the Rc-S* association that could enhance tolerance and make groups more alike. The pre- and posttreatment sessions did tend to increase alcohol tolerance, and this may explain why the impairing effect of alcohol on our tasks in the MR experiments is generally less than that observed in the studies described in Chapter 6.

Fortunately, there are some benefits in assessing pre- and posttreatment effects when R conditions prevail. Because the R condition could only operate to make it difficult to distinguish MR effects on tolerance, their demonstration under such conditions could provide much more compelling evidence of their influence. In addition, the data from the pretreatment session served to check that the impairing effect of the initial dose did not differ among groups, and to measure individual differences in behavioral sensitivity to the dose. The measure of a subject's impairment under the initial dose therefore could be a useful covariate in the analysis of his posttreatment data. Because considerable precision may be gained by adjusting posttreatment scores for initial sensitivity to the dose, covariance analyses have often been employed to assess treatment effects in our MR studies.

## Comparing Mental and Overt Task Practice

Some of our research has tested the tolerance-inducing effect of mentally rehearsing the Rc-S* association under alcohol by comparing its effect with an R and a "rest" treatment (Vogel-Sprott, Rawana, & Webster, 1984). These two treatments were administered as described in Chapter 6. They were included because R had been found to greatly enhance tolerance, and "rest" had little effect. Thus during the treatment sessions, group R performed the task under alcohol with a monetary S* contingent upon the display of Rc. The "rest" group performed the task drug-free with money for maintaining their drug-free level of achievement, and then rested under the dose of alcohol (with no questions asked this time!).

In these experiments, social drinkers learned the pursuit rotor task, and received a pretreatment assessment of the behavioral effect of the alcohol dose when the monetary S* was contingent upon Rc. Six mental or overt performance tests occurred during each of three weekly treatment sessions. The R and MR groups received their tests under alcohol, whereas the "rest" group performed the task for money six times before alcohol was administered on each treatment session. Approximately 1 week after treatment concluded, a fourth drinking session tested posttreatment effects when all groups performed six tests on the task with money (S*) for drug-compensatory performance (Rc).

The initial dose of alcohol produced significant and comparable impairment in all three groups. Therefore, the pretreatment effect of alcohol did not differ among the groups. Figure 12 presents the posttreatment effects. Here a change in performance above the drug-free baseline indicates impairment. A change below the baseline shows performance is better under alcohol than drug-free. The effects of R and "rest" treatments were similar to those obtained in studies described in the previous chapter. Thus significant impairment continued to be displayed after the "rest" treatment, and R treatment had greatly diminished the impairing effect of the dose. The change *below* the baseline displayed by the R group during the posttreatment session shows complete behavioral tolerance.

The result of the MR treatment, of course, is of prime interest. Figure 12 shows it had the same effect as the R treatment. Both mental and overt performance under alcohol that repeatedly associated Rc-S* resulted in complete tolerance to the behavioral effect of the dose.

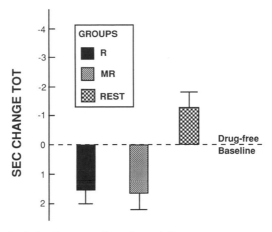

**FIGURE 12.** Alcohol tolerance after three different treatments under alcohol: task performance associating Rc-S* events (group R), mental rehearsal of the association (group MR), or resting ("rest" group). The mean change under alcohol is shown for each group, and a vertical bar shows the *SEM*.

Thus it seemed that environmental and mental events repeating the Rc-S* association had similar tolerance-enhancing effects.

The influence of the MR treatment in this research provided very encouraging support for our hypothesis and prompted additional studies testing other similarities between MR and overt task practice effects on tolerance.

## Mental Rehearsal before or after Alcohol

Our studies of overt task practice, described in Chapter 6, showed that task performance after alcohol only enhanced tolerance if the drug-compensatory response (Rc) was associated with an advantageous consequence (S*). Our R treatment provided an example of this effect. Our studies also included a "rest" treatment that showed drug-free practice before alcohol did not affect tolerance, even though the same desirable S* was administered for performance. From our perspective, a drug-compensatory response, Rc, would only be likely to occur in a drug-related context. The "rest" treatment involved drug-free performance that specifically excluded alcohol, and thus the Rc would be unlikely to occur. Therefore, the "rest" condition appeared to provide no opportunity to relate Rc to any S*, and no information about the consequences of compensating for the effect of alcohol. Thus the ineffectiveness of the "rest" treatment would be attributed to the lack of information about the Rc-S* association. In theory, task performance under alcohol should enhance tolerance only when the occurrence of drug-compensatory performance (Rc) is reliably associated with a favorable S* event. Information about the consequence of compensating for alcohol effects can be learned and provides a Rc-S* expectancy that increases Rc and thereby enhances tolerance.

The explanation of tolerance resulting from overt task practice *before* and *after* alcohol, observed in "rest" and R treatments, respectively, should apply also to mental rehearsal *before* or *after* alcohol. Mental rehearsal of drug-free performance before drinking clearly excludes alcohol effects. With no alcohol-relevant context for mental rehearsal of performance, no compensatory response is likely to be imagined. This would preclude the rehearsal of an Rc-S* association, so no tolerance-inducing Rc-S* expectancy should be acquired. In contrast, mental rehearsal after drinking provides a context relevant to imagining drug-compensatory performance. When the setting also includes a desirable S* for Rc, the association may be rehearsed. Under these conditions, mental rehearsal *after* alcohol should enhance alcohol tolerance to a greater degree than mental rehearsal *before* alcohol.

Some research has tested the alcohol tolerance resulting from mental rehearsal before or after alcohol (Sdao-Jarvie & Vogel-Sprott, 1986). The experiment involved two groups of social drinkers who learned the pursuit rotor, and then received the same dose of alcohol on five weekly drinking sessions. The first and final session provided pre- and posttreatment measures of the effect of the dose when subjects performed the task with a monetary S* contingent upon Rc. During the three intervening sessions, both groups mentally rehearsed the task equally often. One group rehearsed drug-free, *before* drinking alcohol. To reduce the risk that this group might spontaneously mentally rehearse the pursuit rotor task after the dose was received, they performed a series of auditory detection (AD) tasks under alcohol. The AD task required listening and counting but involved no motor activity or any environmental consequence. Thus, in theory, the mental activity of the AD task was unlikely to affect alcohol tolerance. The other group mentally rehearsed pursuit rotor performance *after* alcohol was received. For purposes of control, subjects in this group did the AD tasks before drinking commenced.

The pretreatment dose of alcohol impaired the performance of both groups to a comparable degree. The effect of the dose on the posttreatment session is shown in Figure 13. Changes above the drug-free baseline show that the alcohol still impaired the performance of both groups. However, the effect of the dose was signifi-

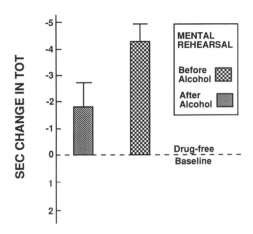

**FIGURE 13.** Tolerance resulting from mental rehearsal before or after alcohol. The mean change under alcohol is shown for each group, and a vertical bar shows the *SEM.*

cantly weaker in the group that mentally rehearsed *after* alcohol was administered. Thus the group with mental practice under alcohol was more tolerant than the group that mentally rehearsed in a drug-free state.

It is important to emphasize that the mental rehearsal was analogous to overt practice under R treatment: Both procedures allowed learning of a desirable S* for drug-compensatory (Rc) performance. In overt performance, S* was a monetary event. In mental performance, the monetary S* was imagined. In theory, the tolerance-inducing effect of both forms of training under alcohol should be due to the S* associated with Rc. In previous chapters, research on overt performance under alcohol showed that tolerance was affected by the presence or absence of S* for Rc. Similar effects should be obtained according to whether when the S* is present or absent in mental practice under alcohol, but our before–after experiment does not address this possibility.

In order to compare the effect of mental rehearsal to the findings on overt performance before and after administration of alcohol, the mental rehearsal study was obligated to adopt a before–after experimental design. However, we have previously noted that evidence from experiments with this design is difficult to interpret. This is because practice after alcohol could involve several factors that might increase tolerance, all of which are absent when practice precedes alcohol. These interpretative problems also apply to our findings on mental rehearsal before or after alcohol. For example, subjects mentally rehearsing after alcohol entered the laboratory for each mental practice trial and sat in front of the task under alcohol. The reliable association of the laboratory task stimuli (S) with the drug (Sd*) could foster a stimulus expectancy for alcohol. More tolerance may have been displayed because these subjects expected alcohol when their task performance was subsequently tested on the posttreatment session. Drug state dependent learning is another possibility. Optimal performance would be expected when training and test conditions occur under the same drug state. The group that mentally rehearsed after alcohol had this advantage because both its treatment and its subsequent test of performance occurred under the drug. The functional demand hypothesis, advanced to account for the effect of overt performance under alcohol, seems unlikely to apply to mental rehearsal under alcohol. Such a hypothesis would have to argue that mental task practice increased functional demands under the drug more than did the control AD activity, and the extra exertion of mental rehearsal somehow increased the tolerance-inducing effect of alcohol.

In summary, the demonstration that mental and overt performance under alcohol can have similar effects on behavioral tolerance contributes an important fact. A hitherto unrecognized factor that may importantly affect the alcohol tolerance of social drinkers has been identified. Moreover, the evidence to this point was encouragingly consistent with the assumption that information about the tolerance-enhancing Rc-S* relationship can be acquired by mental rehearsal of the association. The next section describes experiments designed to test our theoretical explanation of mental rehearsal effects on alcohol tolerance.

## Interpreting Mental Rehearsal Effects

An interpretation of the tolerance-inducing effect of mental rehearsal under alcohol would be greatly aided if we could look inside our subjects' heads to verify their rehearsal of the Rc-S* association. Unfortunately, we cannot tell what they were thinking about, or if they were thinking of anything. Whatever mental activity the subjects were engaged in, we do know that they had repeated doses of alcohol, and the drug effects were always present when subjects were in the laboratory with the task apparatus. The association of alcohol effects with the distinctive task test environment is a classic Pavlovian conditioning procedure for the development of a stimulus expectancy for a drug. Furthermore, the acquisition of such an expectancy has been demonstrated to enhance tolerance. Is it possible that stimulus expectancy could completely explain our results?

Stimulus expectancy could certainly be contributing something to the tolerance we obtained from our mental rehearsal treatment. The crucial question is whether *all* of the tolerance produced could be attributed to stimulus expectancy for alcohol. If the answer is yes, then our theory about specific associations between mental events is unnecessary. Thus one priority for clarifying our interpretation was to separate stimulus expectancy effects from mental rehearsal activity and then determine how much tolerance was attributable to each component.

## Mental Rehearsal in the Same or Different Task Environment

If the association between the task environment and alcohol effects results in a stimulus expectancy that affects tolerance, then the influence of mental rehearsal under alcohol in this environment cannot be distinguished from stimulus expectancy effects. One way to isolate mental rehearsal from stimulus expectancy effects is to conduct mental rehearsal under alcohol in a different setting that excludes the task. This strategy was employed in research that involved four groups of social drinkers (Annear & Vogel-Sprott, 1985). Two groups mentally rehearsed (MR) the pursuit rotor task under alcohol. The rehearsal was similar to our other studies in that it involved imagining performance and its consequence. To control for the possible influence of mental activity under alcohol, two other groups performed an auditory detection (AD) task after drinking. The AD task required listening and counting, but no environmental consequence was associated with task performance and no motor activity was involved.

To associate the expectation of alcohol with the pursuit rotor task, one MR and one AD group received alcohol in the presence of the task. The reliable association between alcohol and the task test environment here presumably could foster a stimulus expectancy for alcohol that should enhance tolerance when the task was performed on the posttreatment alcohol session. The remaining pair of MR and AD groups received their alcohol in an entirely different environment, resembling a library. In the absence of any association between the laboratory task environment and alcohol, stimulus expectancy effects in this pair of groups would be unlikely to occur when the pursuit rotor task was subsequently performed under alcohol.

Pre- and posttreatment measures of the effect of alcohol on

pursuit rotor performance were obtained on the first and the final drinking session. These alcohol test sessions were conducted in an identical fashion for all subjects. The pretreatment effect of alcohol did not differ significantly among the groups. They all displayed a comparable degree of impairment. Figure 14 presents the posttreatment effect of alcohol in each group. Impairment is shown by changes above the drug-free baseline, and more tolerance is indicated by smaller changes that are closer to the baseline.

Mental rehearsal and the environmental setting each affected tolerance. The two groups who had mentally rehearsed the motor task were more tolerant than those who performed auditory detection. The effect of the environment during the posttreatment session showed the groups whose treatment sessions had administered alcohol in a different situation were less tolerant than those who received alcohol in the same environment on all sessions. These posttreatment effects of environment thus are consistent with a tolerance-inducing effect of stimulus expectancy for alcohol. The difference between the MR and AD groups whose treatment under alcohol had occurred in the different environment is of particular interest. The treatment of this pair of groups excluded stimulus expectancy effects on tolerance, because they had had no opportunity to associate alcohol with the task environment in which posttreatment effects were assessed. The superior tolerance of the MR group here shows that mental rehearsal of the Rc-S* association *itself* had a tolerance-enhancing effect. The advantage of combining stimulus expectancy with mental rehearsal is demonstrated by the tolerance of the MR group tested in the same environment. The effect of alcohol on their performance had diminished to such a degree that no

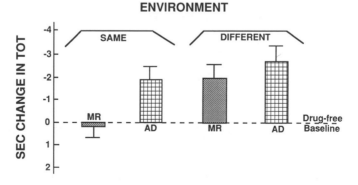

**FIGURE 14.** Tolerance after mental rehearsal in the same or different task environment. The mean change under alcohol is shown for each group, and a vertical bar shows the *SEM*.

impairment was evident. Their posttreatment performance under alcohol was not different from their drug-free level of achievement.

In sum, it appears that our mental rehearsal treatment is a tolerance-inducing phenomenon in its own right. It cannot be due solely to the expectation of alcohol. If the functional demand hypothesis were stretched to cover mental as well as overt activity, it could not explain the results because all subjects performed mental tasks for the same duration under alcohol. State dependent learning also cannot account for the evidence because all subjects performed the task under alcohol on pre- and posttreatment sessions, and the conditions under which they performed were identical. Another explanation is needed.

The added effect of mental rehearsal shown in this research accords with the hypothesis that behavioral tolerance is affected by two learned associations. One is the expectation of receiving alcohol, and the other is the expectation of a desirable consequence for compensating for the drug effect. This latter expectancy is attributed to the reliable association of Rc-S* events. Our evidence implies that this Rc-S* information may be acquired by mental, as well as overt, task practice under alcohol. In theory, this information allows a drinker to expect a desirable consequence for drug-compensatory performance. Such an expectation, in turn, increases the likelihood of displaying compensatory performance (Rc) whenever drinking occurs in the situation. This interpretation implies that the effect of the Rc-S* expectancy acquired during mental rehearsal should be similar to that obtained when Rc-S* events are associated during overt performance. The remainder of this chapter describes research testing some additional predictions concerning mental rehearsal.

## Training History Effects

The evidence examined up to this point suggests that training to associate compensatory performance (Rc) with a favorable consequence (S*) can be accomplished equally well through mental or overt task practice under alcohol. Both modes of training presumably led to an Rc-S* expectancy that enhanced alcohol tolerance to a comparable degree. If this is the case, then a *history* of Rc-S* training, by either mental or overt practice, should produce similar effects. Chapter 6 described some experiments that showed a history of Rc-S* training by overt task practice had enduring effects on alcohol tolerance and response to a placebo. A history of Rc-S* training by mental rehearsal should have similar enduring effects.

The carry-over effect of mental rehearsal training on subsequent tolerance to alcohol and the response to placebo has been tested (Sdao-Jarvie & Vogel-Sprott, in press). This research involved five groups of drinkers who learned the tracometer task and then attended five weekly drinking sessions. Different training was administered to each group during the first three alcohol sessions.

The first alcohol session provided a mental rehearsal (MR) group with the experience of the Rc-S* association that was to be mentally practiced. Thus they performed the tracometer task under alcohol and received a monetary S* contingent upon the display of Rc. During the two remaining training sessions, subjects in the MR group received alcohol and then mentally rehearsed tracometer performance and its outcome. The training administered to the remaining four groups involved overt performance under alcohol. The opportunity to learn the Rc-S* association was provided to two groups (R and I) that performed with a desirable S* reliably contingent upon the display of drug compensatory performance (Rc). The training of the other two groups (M and N) provided no opportunity to learn the Rc-S* association because no S* was related to Rc when they performed under alcohol. These four training treatments were administered in other research (Sdao-Jarvie & Vogel-Sprott, 1991), and were fully described in the section discussing performance and learning effects of the treatments (Chapter 6). All groups received the same number and duration of trials during the three training sessions. Training history effects were assessed on subsequent drinking sessions.

## Tolerance

Approximately 1 week after treatment concluded, a fourth drinking session tested alcohol tolerance. All subjects were advised prior to drinking that they would receive 25 cents for drug-compensatory performance on each test under alcohol, and the monetary S* was dispensed whenever Rc was displayed. Thus all subjects had the same incentive to display Rc during the session. The only difference between the groups resided in their prior training history.

The posttraining tolerance to alcohol was tested on session 4, about a week after training concluded. The effect of alcohol on the performance of each group is shown in Figure 15. Changes above the zero baseline here indicate impairment. Less impairment means a weaker drug effect (i.e, more tolerance). We had previously seen (Chapter 6, Figure 8) that a history of R or I training, in which the Rc-S* association had been trained during overt performance, had an

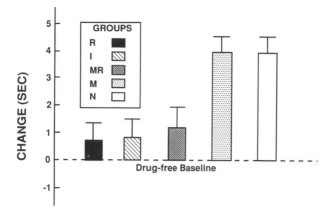

**FIGURE 15.** The effect of a history of mental rehearsal or task practice on performance under alcohol. The mean change under alcohol is shown for each group, and a vertical bar shows the *SEM.*

enduring tolerance-enhancing effect. Theory predicted that a history of training the Rc-S* association by mental rehearsal should have the same effect. In accord with the hypothesis, Figure 15 shows that the tolerance displayed by the group with a history of MR training is comparable to that of the R and I groups who had received overt training. Moreover, the tolerance of these groups is greater than that displayed by the M and N groups whose training history provided no opportunity to acquire the Rc-S* expectancy.

## Response to Placebo

A week after the tolerance test, a fifth drinking session substituted placebo for alcoholic drinks. The session was otherwise exactly identical to the preceding session. Thus all subjects expected alcohol and received the 25-cent S* for displaying drug-compensatory performance. Because alcohol was absent, the session provided an opportunity to test training history effects on an Rc uncontaminated by the effect of alcohol. Insofar as the drug impairs behavior by slowing performance of the task, the compensatory Rc should presumably hasten and facilitate reactions. Thus in the absence of alcohol, Rc should improve performance, so that the task is completed more quickly than normal. In our experiment, this would be shown by a change *below* the zero drug-free level of achievement. The response to placebo, shown in Figure 16, was significantly affected by training history. The groups whose prior training had provided an opportu-

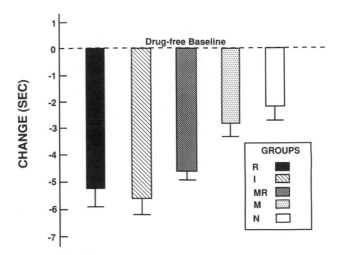

**FIGURE 16.** The effect of a history of mental rehearsal or task practice on the response to a placebo. The mean change under placebo is shown for each group, and a vertical bar shows the *SEM*.

nity to associate Rc with S*, either by performing (R and I) or by mentally rehearsing (MR) under alcohol, continued to show a comparable, and significantly stronger, compensatory reaction under the placebo. Moreover, the intensity of these treatment history effects was a consistent with the degree of alcohol tolerance displayed by the groups in the preceding session (see Figure 15).

The fact that all training groups showed some compensatory facilitation in response to the placebo is also of interest. This tendency could have been fostered, in part, by the tolerance test administered the previous week. The tolerance test had administered a desirable S* for the Rc of all subjects and thus offered the M and N groups an initial opportunity to learn the Rc-S* association. The other factor fostering tolerance in all groups could be a stimulus expectancy for alcohol, acquired because of the repeated administration of alcohol on the preceding four drinking sessions. Both influences could cause the groups to be more alike in their compensatory response to the placebo. However, in spite of these influences, significant group differences attributable to training history were still obtained. Further, the evidence of training history effects was especially compelling because they were detected 2 weeks after the training treatment had concluded.

## A Competing Interpretation of Mental Rehearsal

The robust and reliable effect of our mental rehearsal treatment has been demonstrated sufficiently often that the fact is unlikely now to be questioned. But the evidence implies that mental activity can affect alcohol tolerance, and such a conclusion is far removed from traditional views of tolerance. The conclusion that tolerance can be acquired by mentally rehearsing drug-compensatory performance is likely to be greeted with considerable skepticism. To some, overt task practice under alcohol might seem to offer a more credible explanation, because MR treatment in our experiments was always preceded by one drinking session in which the task was overtly performed under alcohol. Could the effect of mental rehearsal in this research be attributed to the task practice under drug on the first drinking session? This is an important interpretive issue, and merits discussion.

A task practice interpretation of MR effects would note that the MR group performed the task under alcohol with a desirable S* for the display of Rc during its pretraining drinking session 1. Thus its session 1 was identical to that of the group receiving R training. The R training procedure induces considerable tolerance, and it was administered to all groups on the posttraining drinking session. Thus the posttraining tolerance of the MR group, observed when its performance was tested a second time, might be attributed to its task practice under R conditions during the first drinking session. If this interpretation is correct, then the tolerance displayed by the R groups on their second drinking session should be comparable to that of the MR group when their performance under alcohol was tested a second time, on session 4.

The effect of R training on performance under alcohol was measured on each of the four alcohol sessions. The pre- and post-training effects of MR were measured on sessions 1 and 4. Sessions 2 and 3 administered mental rehearsal and, of course, obtained no measures of task performance under alcohol. The effect of the dose on the R group on each of the four sessions is shown in Figure 17, together with the effect observed in the MR group on the pre- and posttraining sessions, 1 and 4. The zero position on the graph represents the drug-free level of achievement on each session, just prior to drinking, and larger positive changes indicate greater impairment under the dose. Both groups were tested for the first time under alcohol on session 1, and Figure 17 shows their impairment did not differ. Their second test occurred on session 2 for group R, and session 4 for group MR. The impairing effect of the alcohol was reduced in both cases, but the groups differed significantly. The MR group was considerably more tolerant. Its performance under alcohol was almost comparable to its drug-free achievement, whereas the R group was still appreciably impaired.

These observations provide strong evidence against the possi-

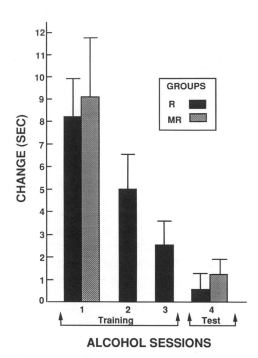

**FIGURE 17.** Alcohol effects during MR or R training (sessions 1–3), and tolerance test session 4. The mean change under alcohol is shown for each group, and a vertical bar shows the *SEM*.

bility that MR treatment effects are due solely to the session 1 task practice under alcohol. MR training clearly had some additional tolerance-inducing effect that was only equaled after three sessions of overt performance under R training.

The results of this research add further evidence consistent with the prediction that mental rehearsal of a task that repeatedly associates imaginary Rc-S* events works just like training where the task is performed and the S* event is contingent upon the display of Rc. Both training procedures enhanced tolerance and led to a strong Rc to a placebo drink when subjects expected alcohol. Yet the evidence concerning the assumption that the repeated mental association of Rc-S* is what causes tolerance is still circumstantial. Skepticism concerning the theoretical interpretation might more readily be allayed by demonstrating that alcohol tolerance is affected by the presence or absence of the imagined consequence of mentally rehearsed performance under drug. In other words, it should be possible to demonstrate that mental rehearsal of task performance *and* its imagined consequence enhances tolerance, whereas identical mental rehearsal of performance with no imagined consequence has little effect on behavioral tolerance to alcohol. The research in the next section is for the skeptics.

## The Imaginary S* in Mental Practice

Our research initially demonstrated that task practice under alcohol very effectively enhanced behavioral tolerance to alcohol if a desirable S* was contingent upon the display of Rc. Therefore, our mental rehearsal treatment was designed to include the Rc-S* association by always asking subjects to evaluate the adequacy of their performance on each imaginary trial. In theory, the tolerance-inducing effect of our mental rehearsal training was attributed to the repeated mental association of the imaginary Rc-S* events. This explanation predicted that mental rehearsal of task performance under alcohol should have little effect on alcohol tolerance if the mental rehearsal does not involve consideration of the desirable outcome of compensatory performance.

Our prediction also appeared relevant to an understanding of mental rehearsal effects during drug-free learning, because it implied that an imagined desirable consequence of a mentally rehearsed task also should improve drug-free performance. Although many learning studies show that the environmental consequence of an overt response will influence its acquisition, little research attention has been paid to the effect of imagined consequences of mentally rehearsed performance. It seems that the phenomenon of mental rehearsal is not well understood (Corbin, 1972; Schmidt, 1988), and there is no clear evidence concerning the effect of imaginary consequences during mental rehearsal of task performance, either drug-free, or under alcohol. To obtain this evidence, two experiments were conducted using the pursuit rotor task. One examined drug-free learning of the task, and the other tested the acquisition of behavioral tolerance to alcohol (Zinatelli & Vogel-Sprott, 1990).

Both experiments involved three treatment groups. One group mentally rehearsed with reminders to evaluate the adequacy of each imaginary practice trial. This treatment represented our customary mental rehearsal procedure, in which imaginary performance was always associated with a consequence. Another group mentally rehearsed with no mention of, or reference to, the outcome of performance. Thus this group had equal practice imagining task performance, but with no associated consequence. A third group served as control and rested while the other groups had mental rehearsal trials. Treatment effects were evaluated by a pre- and a posttraining test of pursuit rotor performance, conducted under identical conditions for all groups.

The drug-free experiment examined treatment effects on the acquisition of pursuit rotor skill. In the experiment on alcohol tolerance, subjects learned the task drug-free, and the treatments were subsequently administered under repeated doses of alcohol. Both experiments found mental rehearsal with imaginary consequences to yield the most powerful effects, enhancing drug-free achievement and alcohol tolerance more than did either mental rehearsal without imaginary consequences, or resting (Zinatelli & Vogel-Sprott, 1990).

Our theoretical explanation of the tolerance-enhancing effect of mental rehearsal under alcohol attributed it to the reliable association of imaginary performance with a desirable consequence, Rc-S*. The explanation was confirmed. Tolerance was enhanced when mental rehearsal involved the Rc-S* association, and mental rehearsal without the S* had a minimal effect. Additional support in principle for this explanation was provided by the effect of drug-free mental rehearsal on the acquisition of a motor skill. Here too, mental rehearsal that associated imagined performance with S* was the most beneficial. Together the findings suggest that the S* during mental rehearsal may be a generally important ingredient that determines the efficacy of mental rehearsal. Even more generally, the results are in accord with the literature on instrumental learning that also indicates that the consequences of a response will affect its display.

## Can Mental Rehearsal without Alcohol Induce Tolerance?

Research described up to this point has used an Rc-S* training procedure to induce tolerance, and compared the effect of administering the training by mental or overt task practice. Both modes of training included the four events that our analysis predicted would affect tolerance. The theory was presented in Chapter 4, and Figure 3B identified the events as:

| S ⟶ | Sd ⟶ | Rc ⟶ | S* |
|---|---|---|---|
| stimulus cues predicting drug | drug stimulus | compensatory response | desirable outcome |

The training by mental and overt task practice was considered to differ only with respect to the nature of the Rc-S* events. Mental training required imagination, so that the Rc-S* association was cognitively rehearsed. In contrast, overt practice associated the actual events, Rc-S*; no imagination was involved. Nonetheless, the two modes of training were comparable in many respects. A reliable Rc-S* association enhanced tolerance whether the relationship was rehearsed mentally or by overt task practice. In addition, both forms of training were only effective if they were conducted in an alcohol-related context, and a favorable S* was associated with Rc. Equivalent training in a drug-free situation had little effect on alcohol tolerance, even when a desirable S* was provided for Rc. Because drug-free task performance specifically excludes the alcohol (Sd*) event from the situation, the absence of Sd* eliminates the relevance of a drug-compensatory response, Rc. Thus, in theory, the drug-free situation would be unlikely to involve any real or imaginary Rc, so no information about the tolerance-enhancing Rc-S* association would be provided.

One means of ensuring the presence of the Sd* is to conduct training when the drug has been administered. Our training of subjects under doses of alcohol served this purpose. However, the actual administration of alcohol may not be the only way of ensuring an alcohol-related context for the training. After a drinker has an experience performing a task under alcohol, the impairing effect of alcohol might be imagined when the individual is in a drug-free state. Spontaneously, or under instruction, a person may imagine the effect of alcohol and mentally rehearse task performance and its outcome. In other words, the entire experience is imagined. This instance of mental rehearsal would involve three imagined events: the drug stimulus (Sd*), a compensatory response (Rc), and a favorable outcome (S*). All our previous MR treatments only required subjects to imagine Rc and S*. The addition of the imagined drug stimulus (Sd*) could presumably create an alcohol-related context for the training without actually administering the drug. Thus we come to a most novel hypothesis: A drug-free treatment in which drinkers mentally rehearse the imaginary alcohol effect (Sd), ensuing compensatory performance (Rc), and its desirable consequence (S*) should enhance behavioral tolerance to alcohol. The proposal that alcohol tolerance can be enhanced in the absence of concomitant drug use could not be predicted by any prevailing theory of drug tolerance. Indeed, it would probably be an understatement to say that our prediction is counterintuitive. Yet such a drug-free mental rehearsal treatment bears a close resemblance to a widely used clinical cognitive therapy technique that trains a patient to mentally rehearse coping responses in the presence of some imaginary disrupting stimulus that had previously been experienced (Meichenbaum, 1977).

Several of our experiments have tested the behavioral tolerance to alcohol resulting from mentally rehearsing performance while imagining alcohol effects (MRIA). This MRIA treatment required subjects in a drug-free state to imagine the drug effect (Sd*), the compensatory response (Rc), and its outcome (S*). The studies have compared the tolerance obtained from MRIA treatment with two other treatment procedures. One was mental rehearsal (MR) under alcohol. Here the compensatory response and its outcome are imagined under doses of alcohol, so the drug stimuli (Sd*) are actually present. The studies we have already reviewed show that this MR training reliably yields a high degree of alcohol tolerance. The other condition was a "rest" treatment that equated the doses of alcohol the MR group received, but involved no mental rehearsal. Our other studies have shown that the "rest" condition tends to have negligible effects on tolerance. The inclusion of MR and "rest" groups in our experiments provided a means of estimating of the maximum and minimum effects, respectively, that could be observed. Thus, by comparing the tolerance resulting from MRIA to that obtained from MR and "rest," the experiments could locate the effect of the MRIA within the range of possible effects. Treatment sessions intervened between a pretreatment alcohol session and the posttreatment session. On the pre- and posttreatment sessions, all groups performed a pursuit rotor task under alcohol with a monetary S* contingent upon drug-compensatory performance (Rc).

The pretreatment sessions in our experiments obtained no significant group differences in the impairing effect of the dose. Thus, prior to the onset of the treatments, the drug effect was comparable in all groups. The posttreatment effects in these studies have yielded consistent results, and a summary of the effects is presented in Figure 18. Group MR, whose training had consisted of mentally rehearsing the task under alcohol, no longer displayed any impairment under the dose. Of course, these results were predicted on the basis of our other experiments showing that MR treatment yields a high degree of tolerance. Also in accordance with our prior findings, the "rest" group continued to display a significant degree of impairment and gave little evidence of tolerance. The MRIA treatment is of major interest, and our experiments have repeatedly found it yielded intermediate effects. Our drug-free MRIA treatment resulted in *less* tolerance than MR where the drug effects did not have to be imagined, and *more* tolerance than resting under repeated doses of

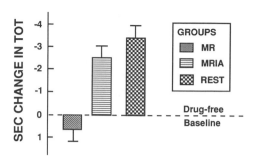

FIGURE 18. Alcohol effects after groups had mentally rehearsed under alcohol (MR), mentally rehearsed under imaginary alcohol effects (MRIA), or rested under alcohol ("rest"). The mean change under alcohol is shown for each group, and a vertical bar shows the *SEM.*

alcohol. Figure 18 also shows that the actual size of the effect of MRIA treatment is small, and in each of our experiments the MRIA and "rest" groups failed to differ significantly.

During debriefings, the MRIA subjects in our experiments reported that they could fairly readily imagine the drug stimuli (Sd*) or task performance and its consequence (Rc-S*), but it was extremely difficult to imagine *both* simultaneously. However, many subjects thought that this could be achieved with more practice. Because an experiment required subjects to participate for 6 weeks, extending the study by adding more weeks of treatment was not feasible. Thus our experiments were repeated using several different techniques to increase the effect of MRIA treatment within a 6-week period. Giving subjects cassette recordings of the mental rehearsal instructions to play and rehearse daily at home was one promising technique that was tried. In total, five experiments were conducted, each using a different procedure that appeared likely to provide more MRIA training. In every case, the effect of this treatment fell in an intermediate position, between MR and "rest." Whereas the probability of reproducing this ordering of group means five times in succession is <0.001, the actual size of the difference between the MRIA and "rest" groups has only attained a probability level of 0.14. It seems then, that MR under imaginary alcohol effects may generate some tolerance, but within the constraints of an experiment only marginal effects are likely to be evident.

In real-world situations, alcohol tolerant behavior can have many advantageous outcomes, such as avoiding fatal accidents, criminal charges, fines, or imprisonment. These outcomes are surely more desirable than the small monetary rewards that could be used in our experiments. Social drinkers also could mentally rehearse drug-compensatory performance under imaginary alcohol effects during months or years, a period of practice that cannot be matched in any experiment. The results of our experiments with mental rehearsal under imaginary alcohol effects are not conclusive. Yet they do prompt the speculation that if experiments could be conducted using real-world consequences and months of training, this drug-free treatment may indeed induce behavioral tolerance to alcohol.

## Summary

This chapter reviewed research on the effect of mental rehearsal on behavioral tolerance to alcohol. Social drinkers received a pre- and a posttreatment session in which they performed a task under alcohol with a desirable consequence (S*) contingent upon drug compensatory performance (Rc). Mental rehearsal training was administered on intervening drinking sessions and consisted of repeated trials under alcohol in which task performance and its outcome (Rc-S*) were imagined.

The effects of mental rehearsal treatment were found to be essentially similar to training the Rc-S* association through overt performance under alcohol. Thus both procedures resulted in a comparable degree of tolerance to alcohol and generated a strong compensatory response (Rc) to a placebo when alcohol was expected. Many conditions determining the efficacy of the two treatments were also similar. In both cases, a reliable Rc-S* relationship was necessary because training that excluded the S* so that there was no Rc-S* association had little effect on tolerance. In addition, both training procedures had to be administered in an alcohol-related context. Equivalent mental or overt task practice in a drug-free state was ineffective.

The two training procedures were also more effective when training occurred in the specific task environment in which tolerance was subsequently tested. However, the evidence also suggested that mental rehearsal might be more portable because it could induce tolerance when the mental training was administered in a situation where the task was physically absent. In addition, some suggestive evidence indicated that mental rehearsal of the task while just imaging the alcohol effect could induce some tolerance.

The tolerance-inducing effect of the mental and overt task training was attributed to the acquisition of information concerning the reliable association between drug-compensatory performance (Rc) and a desirable consequence (S*). The retention of this information allowed drinkers to expect this consequence for compensating for the alcohol effect. Thus the effect of both procedures was considered to rest upon the learning of this Rc-S* expectancy. The findings on mental rehearsal were predicted by our learning analysis of alcohol tolerance and apparently cannot be predicted or explained by other theories of alcohol tolerance.

Our investigations of tolerance in terms of a compensatory response are consistent with the general assumption that tolerance involves a drug compensation reaction. However, the reaction is customarily assumed to be induced by the action of the drug, and our research demonstrates that environmental or mental events associated with a response to a drug can affect behavioral tolerance in a fashion predictable by instrumental learning principles. Because the evidence was based upon studies of social drinkers, the findings identify a hitherto neglected determinant of the alcohol tolerance they could acquire during a social drinking career. To the extent that alcohol tolerance poses a risk of alcohol abuse, it seems that a drinker's learning history may have an equal or more important role to play than the pharmacological effect of the doses of alcohol used by social drinkers.

# V

**EXPECTANCY
EFFECTS
DURING A
SINGLE DOSE**

# 8

## Acute Alcohol Tolerance

It is convenient for a theory to use abstract symbols, such as Rc-S*, to represent the association of drug-compensatory performance with an advantageous consequence. But such an association can be found in many real-world drinking situations. One example could be a drinking driver who is stopped in a police spot check. Our theory applied to this situation would consider the first encounter to provide an ideal opportunity to learn that drug-compensatory performance is advantageous. This response–outcome association would likely be implied upon entering the situation. Confirming information also should accumulate with time, as the suspect performs roadside tests for police appraisal. The reliable information should result in an increasingly certain expectation of the beneficial outcome of compensating for alcohol effects. The occurrence of compensatory behavior should increase and greater resistance to the effect of alcohol should be displayed. By the time the police interview concludes, the drinking driver may appear quite sober, displaying much less or no behavioral effects of alcohol.

The police spot check is an example of a single drinking situation in which information about the advantageous consequence of compensating for alcohol effects is likely to be very frequently repeated. In learning terms, the situation could be viewed as administering a huge number of Rc-S* training trials during a single dose of alcohol. The research on tolerance to repeated doses of alcohol, described in previous chapters, administered analogous, but comparatively few, trials under a dose. The small number of trials might explain why our various training conditions usually did not affect alcohol tolerance until after the first dose and more training trials had occurred.

However, given sufficient information, a drinker should acquire an Rc-S* expectancy during a single dose. The acquisition of the expectancy should be a function of time after drinking, as trials conveying this information accumulate. Thus the influence of the expectancy in enhancing resistance to impairment would likely be strongest during the declining phase of the blood alcohol curve. Such an effect could produce a phenomenon resembling *acute tolerance* to a single dose of alcohol. The essential defining characteristic of acute tolerance is that the effect of alcohol at a particular BAC is more intense on the rising than on the falling limb of the blood alcohol curve.

This chapter presents evidence on the changing pattern of impairment under a dose of alcohol as drinkers acquire information about the Rc-S* association. The effect of this learning on acute tolerance is an important consideration in these studies. Thus a framework for understanding our experimental design and measures requires some discussion of the methodology in past research on acute tolerance.

## Background

Some early findings on acute tolerance were briefly mentioned in Chapter 1. Acute tolerance was first reported by Mellanby (1919), who examined the gait of dogs under a dose of alcohol. While BAC was rising, he measured the BAC at the first observable onset of impairment. During the declining limb of the BAC curve, he measured the BAC associated with recovery (i.e., when impairment was no longer evident). He found that the BAC threshold for recovery from the drug effect was typically higher than the onset threshold. The consistent occurrence of a higher BAC for the recovery from alcohol-induced impairment was subsequently confirmed in the performance of a variety of tasks by humans whose drinking habits ranged from light to very heavy (Goldberg, 1943).

Goldberg's (1943) research was of particular interest because it also showed that the BAC thresholds for the appearance and disappearance of drug effects varied with the type of task and with drinking habits. Compared with light drinkers, extremely heavy drinkers were generally less susceptible to alcohol. They attained higher BAC thresholds for the onset *and* the recovery from impairment in task performance. This finding has probably tended to encourage the assumption that greater use and exposure to alcohol is responsible for enhancing resistance to its effects and accelerating the recovery of function during declining BAC. However, such a finding is open to many other interpretations because there is no way of knowing whether the greater acute tolerance displayed by very heavy drinkers preceded their high alcohol consumption, or caused it, or developed because of some other factor during their drinking careers.

The detection of BAC thresholds for the onset and recovery from the behavioral effect of a dose of alcohol usually requires repeated testing of performance. This led Goldberg (1943) and others (Carpenter, 1962) to suggest that the repeated tests could provide practice under alcohol that may introduce learning and improve performance. These learning effects would become stronger with practice, and this would be correlated with time under the dose. Thus it appeared that the threshold measure indicating accelerated recovery during declining BAC might simply be a learning artifact. In addition, other investigators (Harger & Forney, 1963) questioned the accuracy of BAC measures from the blood samples used in early studies of acute tolerance. Together these doubts seem to have discouraged research on acute tolerance for some decades. With better technology to assess BAC, and a more congenial breath sampling procedure for humans, interest revived and a different measure was devised to test the existence of acute tolerance as a phenomenon in its own right.

Instead of assessing acute tolerance by the threshold BACs for the onset and recovery of the effect of alcohol, experiments measured and compared the behavioral effect induced by a particular BAC on each limb of the blood alcohol curve. These latter measures allowed experiments to be designed to exclude or control task practice effects. For example, two groups of subjects could receive a dose of alcohol, and each could be tested at a given BAC on one of the limbs of the blood alcohol curve. Because each group would only be tested once under alcohol, the measures excluded practice effects. Other experimental designs could control task practice effects by testing one group twice at a particular BAC on each limb of the curve, and administering equivalent tests to a placebo control group. Experiments of this sort have also revealed acute tolerance in a variety of tasks performed by animals and humans (Hurst & Bagley, 1972; LeBlanc, Gibbins, & Kalant, 1975a; Vogel-Sprott, 1979).

Studies of acute tolerance when task practice is excluded or controlled show that the phenomenon is not a complete artifact of task practice. But such studies, of course, cannot tell us whether learning may affect acute tolerance. Although that question remains open, the findings have often been considered to indicate that learning has no role to play, and acute tolerance likely reflects adaptation to the pharmacological action of alcohol that develops with time during the course of a dose.

The assumption that acute tolerance is due to a single adaptive process implies that the amount of acute tolerance displayed by an individual should be consistent. Yet Goldberg (1943) found that the amount of acute tolerance a drinker displayed varied on different tasks, and appeared to depend upon task familiarity. In addition, research has shown that the same individual, performing two tasks alternately at comparable BACs, can display pronounced acute tolerance on one task, and no vestige of acute tolerance on another (Vogel-Sprott, 1979).

It seems that within-subject variability in acute tolerance cannot be explained by assuming a single adaptive mechanism is at work during exposure to a dose of alcohol. Nonetheless, little attention has been given to individual inconsistencies in the display of acute tolerance. The neglect may be due, in part, to the fact that research in the area has been preoccupied with demonstrating that acute tolerance is not solely attributable to learning under alcohol. This work has been based upon the assumption that the amount of task practice under alcohol directly determines the learning that affects acute tolerance. However, it now appears that this assumption is incorrect. Our experiments on tolerance to repeated doses of alcohol showed task practice per se did not necessarily involve the learning needed to induce tolerance. The learning that affected tolerance depended upon the *consequence* of task performance. The research described in this chapter pursues this hypothesis with respect to acute tolerance and the profile of impairment under a dose of alcohol.

## Measurement of Acute Tolerance

The best way to relate the findings of our research on acute tolerance to the results of others is to use the same criterion measure. Prior experiments have commonly identified acute tolerance by measuring BAC thresholds for the onset and recovery from the effect of the dose, or by calculating the intensity of the behavioral effect of a given BAC on each limb of the alcohol curve.

Contemporary research on acute tolerance has favored the technique of measuring the drug effect twice, at the same BAC on each limb of the alcohol curve. The reliability of detecting acute tolerance by this procedure has received little consideration or discussion. Moreover, there are some difficulties in using this measure to assess the acute tolerance of social drinkers. Tests of the behavioral effects of alcohol on social drinkers are usually based upon moderate doses that yield peak BACs near 80 mg/100 ml, and acute tolerance is often tested by selecting a criterion BAC in the range of 50–70 mg/100 ml.

The decision about the BAC at which to test performance must be made prior to the experiment. The choice of an adequate BAC criterion requires considerable information about the typical effect of alcohol on a task during a dose. This is illustrated in Figure 19, which shows rising and declining BACs in the 50–70 mg/100 ml range, and the associated percent impairment in performance likely to be displayed on the motor skill tasks in our alcohol experiments. The A positions on the curve of impairment in the figure show a 15% degradation of performance is obtained at a BAC of 70 mg/100 ml on each limb of the curve. If this BAC criterion were used, comparisons would lead to the conclusion that no acute tolerance occurred. But suppose a criterion of 60 mg/100 ml were employed, shown by the B positions in the figure. Acute tolerance here would be demonstrated because this BAC yields 8% impairment on the rising limb of the alcohol curve, and 0% impairment on the declining limb. The C positions in the figure represent the adoption of a 50 mg/100 ml BAC criterion. The evidence here would yield another different result. Because no impairment on the task is displayed at a BAC of 50/100 ml on either limb of the alcohol curve, an investigator would conclude that task performance is not impaired by alcohol. The comparatively narrow range of testable BACs makes the selection appear trivial, but a narrow scope of BACs does not necessarily mean that the intensity of the drug effect also has a small range. The success in detecting

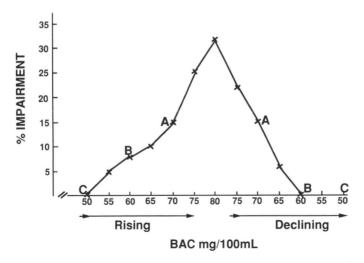

**FIGURE 19.** Conclusions concerning acute tolerance depend upon the BAC selected for comparison on the two limbs of the alcohol curve.

acute tolerance can hinge critically on the selection of the criterion BAC, even within a seemingly restricted range.

Figure 19 illustrates how three entirely different conclusions could be obtained from the same data when only two measures are obtained at arbitrarily chosen BACs. The example only concerns cases where moderate doses of alcohol are administered, but it is likely to apply to most research with social drinkers. Here the important point is that misleading conclusions may be obtained when acute tolerance is only assessed at a selected BAC on each limb of the BAC curve.

The other common measure of acute tolerance is based on BAC thresholds for the onset and for recovery from the effect of a dose. It requires frequent, regular assessment of the behavioral effect of the dose. The BAC thresholds are identified by the first test that detects a drug effect, and by the first test thereafter that detects no effect of the drug. In Figure 19, a BAC of 55 mg/100 ml would identify the appearance threshold because it is the first test during rising BAC that reveals impairment. The recovery threshold during declining BAC is identified by the first test that shows a return to the drug-free level of achievement, that is, 0% impairment. This occurs at a BAC of 60 mg/100 ml. These BAC thresholds reveal acute tolerance because performance returns to normal at a declining BAC that is higher than needed to impair performance when blood alcohol levels are rising.

Because the determination of BAC thresholds involves regular assessments of the drug effect during the course of a dose, threshold measures insure that *any* acute tolerance that is displayed will be detected. Thus this procedure is less likely to result in misleading conclusions that could arise when only two measures of the drug effect are obtained at a given BAC on each limb of the alcohol curve. Nonetheless, BAC threshold measures are thought to have a rather limited utility. In part, this opinion is based upon the correct recognition that they can only be obtained with a behavior that has a well-defined, stable characteristic *prior* to the administration of alcohol. A stable drug-free baseline is required in order to detect the onset and recovery from the alcohol-induced change in behavior. Of course, a stable level of performance is only likely to be obtained on tasks with which subjects are familiar before alcohol is administered. If the task is one that subjects could have learned or performed under alcohol prior to the experiment, then uncontrolled individual differences in task familiarity could contaminate the evidence. Therefore, many experimenters choose to measure alcohol effects on the performance of a novel task that subjects perform for the first time under the drug. BAC thresholds cannot be measured in such studies because no prior stable drug-free criterion of a subject's performance is available. But the limitation is imposed more by the experimental design than by the BAC threshold measures. If experiments using novel tasks included a drug-free practice period prior to the dose of alcohol, this preliminary practice could control individual differences in prior learning of a task and would provide a stable baseline measure of performance for the evaluation of subsequent alcohol effects.

A greater impediment to measuring BAC thresholds likely stems from the view that the repeated performance of a task under alcohol needed to identify the thresholds introduces learning effects that contaminate the assessment of acute tolerance. However, our theory and research on tolerance suggest this opinion is misguided. The frequency of task practice under alcohol, does not, by itself, necessarily involve the learning that influences tolerance. The important consideration is the *consequence* of task performance under alcohol.

Acute tolerance in contemporary research is usually measured by comparing drug effects at a given BAC on each limb of the curve. This method is likely popular because it can control task practice effects and can be applied whether or not a task has been well learned prior to receiving alcohol. Nonetheless, BAC threshold measures have the potential to yield more trustworthy information upon which to base conclusions about the display of acute alcohol tolerance by social drinkers. For this reason, our research chose to assess acute tolerance by BAC thresholds.

The decision to use BAC thresholds required preliminary research to develop and test a threshold criterion that could reliably identify a change in the normal performance of a task. The task had to be unfamiliar to subjects prior to an experiment, so that individual differences in prior learning of the task and the experience of alcohol on task performance could be controlled. The pursuit rotor and tracometer tasks are suitable in these respects because subjects have no opportunity to perform these tasks before they enter an experiment.

Haubenreisser (1985) developed the criterion needed for our experiments. His strategy was to provide a few days of drug-free training on the motor skill task, until a set of several consecutive trials showed no significant change. Thus, in terms of a statistical test, the scores on these trials were essentially equivalent indicators of a subject's stable level of drug-free achievement. The mean and the standard deviation *(SD)* of the scores a subject obtained on these trials identified the range of scores a subject was likely to obtain when the task was performed drug-free. For example, scores within ±1 *SD* of a subject's mean would likely be attained 68% of the time the task was performed. Scores greater than $+1$ $SD$ above the mean represented poorer performance while better achievement was indicated by scores $-1$ $SD$ below the mean. Thus the use of the mean and $SD$ of a subject's drug-free scores served to specify the boundaries of his normal drug-free performance and to identify a change in performance by scores outside the range.

Haubenreisser (1985) determined that test scores exceeding $+1$ $SD$ of a subject's mean drug-free score provided a criterion that reliably identified the BAC threshold for the onset of impairment. The criterion was tested by administering a dose of alcohol to drinkers who then performed the task at regular intervals. Subjects' BACs were measured each time the task was performed. The first trial score that was $+1$ $SD$ above a subject's drug-free mean score identified the onset of impairment. This was always observed during the rising limb of the alcohol curve. When the first indication of impairment was displayed, a subject continued to obtain scores $+1$ $SD$ above his mean on subsequent tests during rising alcohol levels. The BAC threshold for recovery was identified by the first test score that reentered the normal range (i.e., differed by less than $+1$ $SD$ from the drug-free mean). Recovery was always observed while BACs were declining, and subsequent scores also remained within the drug-free range. Additional tests of the criterion when drinkers performed under a placebo showed that performance did not improve significantly and that a subject's test scores did not exceed the $\pm 1$ $SD$ range of the drug-free scores.

Our research measured acute tolerance using Haubenreisser's criteria for BAC thresholds for the onset and recovery from the effect of a dose of alcohol. These studies tested the prediction that resistance to the behavioral effect of a dose of alcohol increases as a function of accumulating Rc-S* training, that is, trials conveying information about the favorable consequence of drug-compensatory performance. Thus the effect of the training should be most pronounced during the declining phase of the BAC curve.

## Acquisition Affects Acute Tolerance

In previous chapters, our studies on repeated doses of alcohol evaluated the effect of each dose by the mean change in performance on several trials that occurred at intervals after drinking. Experiments that administered six Rc-S* training trials under each dose typically obtained strong tolerance after three or four drinking sessions. Thus it appeared that the accumulation of 18 to 24 such training trials under a single dose of alcohol should provide sufficiently reliable information to result in an Rc-S* expectancy that increases the occurrence of Rc and enhances resistance to the effect of alcohol. The administration of this number of trials takes time. When trials all occur after drinking a single dose of alcohol, the accumulation of trials is correlated with time under the dose. Therefore, the resistance to impairment resulting from acquiring an Rc-S* expectancy during a dose of alcohol should be strongest during the declining phase of the blood alcohol curve. Here it should operate to enhance acute tolerance, raising the threshold BAC for recovery from the effect of a dose of alcohol and shortening the total duration of impairment.

Experiments have tested this hypothesis by measuring the BAC thresholds for the onset and recovery from the impairing effect of a dose of alcohol on tracometer performance (Haubenreisser & Vogel-Sprott, 1987). Each experiment involved two groups of subjects who received extensive drug-free training on the task to establish a baseline level of achievement. To acquaint subjects with the treatment conditions they would receive under alcohol, an additional day of drug-free practice was administered. Subjects in group R received a monetary S* for maintaining their drug-free level of performance, and the other group (N) received no S* for their task performance. The introduction of the S* to the R group at this late stage of drug-free training did not affect their performance. The task scores of the two groups did not differ and did not change significantly over the set of trials. Subjects took an average of 141 seconds to complete a tracometer trial. A subject's mean drug-free score ±1 SD was used to identify the range of scores equivalent to his drug-free performance, and subjects' SD's ranged from 1.6 to 5.0 seconds.

A dose of alcohol was administered on a subsequent day. A total of 20 trials on the tracometer were administered during a 3-hour period after drinking commenced. The first trial occurred 15 minutes after drinking began, and six trials were completed during the first 60 minutes. The remaining 14 trials were performed at regular intervals thereafter. BAC was measured at periodic intervals and whenever the onset and recovery from alcohol effects were displayed. During the rising BAC, the first test score that was slower by more than +1 SD beyond a subject's drug-free mean score identified the BAC threshold for the onset of impairment. The first test score that reentered the +1 SD range identified the BAC threshold for recovery.

The two groups were treated differently only with respect to the consequence of their performance under alcohol. The group R subjects received a monetary S* contingent upon the display of Rc.

Thus their trials provided an opportunity to acquire the Rc-S*
expectancy. The N group performed the task equally often under the
dose, but no S* was administered for their performance. These R and
N treatments were identical to those described in previous chapters
on tolerance to repeated doses of alcohol.

The effect of R and N training on BAC thresholds, and the times
they were observed during the drinking session are shown in Figure
20. In these experiments, a mean peak BAC of 72 mg/100 ml was
obtained 70 minutes after drinking began. During rising BACs, the
onset of impairment in group N was observed on the second trial.
This trial was performed 20 minutes after drinking commenced, when
the BAC averaged 24 mg/100 ml. The onset of impairment in group R
was detected on the fifth trial, 50 minutes into the session and when
the mean rising BAC was 54 mg/100 ml. Figure 20 also shows that
recovery during the declining limb of the alcohol curve was observed
sooner and at a higher BAC in group R than in group N. The
performance of the group R had recovered to their drug-free level of
proficiency by the 11th trial, when their declining BAC was 63 mg/100
ml. In contrast, recovery in group N was only detected on trial 15,
when BAC had declined to 48 mg/100 ml. The greater resistance of the
R group to the alcohol effect also dramatically reduced the total
duration of their impairment. Figure 20 shows that the period from
the onset to recovery from impairment in group R spanned 70
minutes, as compared with 160 minutes in the N group.

The higher BAC threshold for recovery and overall shorter
duration of impairment under R training are consistent with the

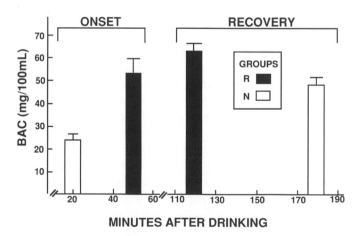

**FIGURE 20.** Mean *(SEM)* BAC thresholds for the onset and recovery from
impairment during a dose of alcohol in groups receiving R or N training.

prediction that reliable information about the favorable consequence of drug-compensatory performance will enhance acute tolerance. R training also increased resistance to the onset of impairment during rising BACs. Because this effect was obtained after only five R training trials during the early rising BAC, it seems that we had underestimated the number of trials needed to acquire an influential Rc-S* expectancy. Drinkers were smarter than we thought. Yet the superior resistance to impairment, displayed by the R group during *both* the rising and the declining limbs of the alcohol curve raised a potential interpretive problem: These same results could have been obtained if subjects in the R groups had been more resistant to alcohol at the *outset* of the experiment, before any trials were performed. Such a bias in the assignment of subjects to the R treatment seemed unlikely because drinkers had been randomly assigned to groups and the experiment had been replicated. Nonetheless, the research provided no means of demonstrating that the effect of alcohol was comparable in the groups *before* they received their treatments. We need another experiment to clarify our interpretation of the effect of R training trials on the onset of impairment.

If R trials during very early rising BACs explain the heightened threshold for the onset of impairment, then this effect should weaken when R trials are delayed, and only begin after somewhat higher rising BACs (e.g., 40 mg/100 ml) are attained. This evidence was obtained in another study that measured BAC thresholds for onset and recovery and the amount of impairment displayed at specific BACs on the blood alcohol curve (Vogel-Sprott, Kartechner, & McConnell, 1989). The research employed Haubenreisser's criterion for the onset and recovery from impairment, and subjects also performed 20 trials on the task after drinking commenced. In order to measure impairment at rising and declining BACs of 40, 50, 60, and 70 mg/100 ml, four of the trials were scheduled with respect to a subject's BAC, and the remainder were administered at temporal intervals. Under this procedure, subjects only performed one trial during early rising BACs of less than 40 mg/100 ml. The study involved four treatment groups. Two groups had training trials that fostered the learning of the Rc-S* association. The training of these two "learning" groups was identical in that a favorable S* was contingent upon the display of Rc. But one group received a monetary S*, whereas the other received an informative S* without any money. These two treatments were identified, respectively, as R and I in preceding chapters, where they were described. In theory, these two training conditions would be considered as cheap and expensive forms of the same training. The trials of the remaining two groups provided no opportunity to learn an Rc-S* association. These "no-learning" groups performed the task after drinking with no S* event reliably associated with Rc. Their treatments were described in previous chapters and identified as RR and N. The RR group received the same number of monetary rewards that were administered during the expensive learning training, but the money was administered randomly with respect to Rc. This expensive no-learning treatment thus provided a monetary incentive to perform the task, but the money was not related to compensatory performance. The other no-learning group (N) had no money, information, or other S* event contingent upon task performance. This latter group obviously received a cheap form of no-learning treatment.

There were no significant group differences in the BAC thresholds for the onset of impairment. This result thus differs from our previous experiment with Haubenreisser where group differences in the onset thresholds were obtained. But that study also administered many more trials during early rising BACs. Thus the results now obtained could be due to too few trials while the BAC was rising. In accord with this interpretation, the effect of accumulating trials became evident by the time BAC started to decline. Here the BAC recovery threshold of the learning groups was significantly higher than that of the no-learning groups. In addition, the recovery thresholds under cheap (no money) and expensive (money) forms of each type of treatment did not differ significantly. This indicated that there was no main effect of money per se. The higher BAC recovery threshold under the learning treatment also resulted in a significantly shorter duration of impairment under the dose. The mean period of impairment in the learning condition was 52 minutes, as compared to 112 minutes in the no-learning condition.

A similar pattern of effects was demonstrated in the measures of the intensity of impairment during rising and declining BACs. When the task was performed at rising BACs of 50, 60, and 70 mg/100 ml, the groups did not differ significantly. However, performance at declining BACs of 60, 50, and 40 mg/100 ml showed the learning treatment resulted in significantly less impairment than the No Learning treatment. The treatment effects are illustrated in Figure 21 where the measures of impairment at 50 and 60 mg/100 ml are averaged to show the effects at mean rising and declining BACs of 55 mg/100 ml.

The only difference between the learning and no-learning conditions in the experiment was the presence or absence of information about the desirable consequence for drug-compensatory performance. Thus the information apparently raised the BAC threshold for

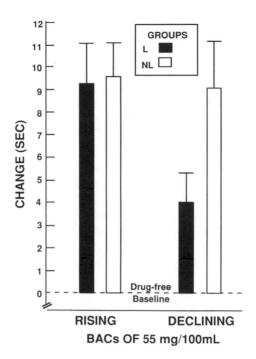

**FIGURE 21.** Mean *(SEM)* impairment at rising and declining BACs of 55 mg/100ml in groups receiving learning (L) or no-learning (NL) training.

recovery from impairment and thereby shortened the duration of the drug effect. In theory, reliable information about the Rc-S* associa-tion should accumulate with repeated trials and allow the acquisition of a more certain and influential Rc-S* expectancy. This expectancy should increase the occurrence of Rc and thus enhance resistance to the impairing effect of alcohol.

In summary, these findings are consistent with the prediction that the effect of learning the Rc-S* association should become stronger as training trials accumulate. Evidence of these effects during a single dose of alcohol adds some new insight and perspec-tives on the phenomenon of acute tolerance. It appears that earlier investigators' suspicions that learning may affect acute tolerance were well founded. But this concern tended to bias the focus of research, so investigations primarily aimed to determine that acute tolerance was a phenomenon in its own right, and not a learning artifact. Thus, because learning was thought to depend upon task practice under alcohol, the solution was to assess acute tolerance in experiments that excluded or controlled task practice. This approach certainly set the learning factor aside, but it also provided no information on whether or how learning affects acute tolerance. Our research contributes some answers to these questions. The evidence shows that task practice under alcohol per se does not necessarily enhance acute tolerance. The activity of performing a task is only important insofar as it provides an opportunity to acquire information about the desirable consequence of compensating for the behavioral effect of the drug. Studies of acute tolerance have aimed to control learning effects by controlling the frequency of task practice under alcohol without regard to the consequence of performance under the drug. Most studies of acute tolerance in animals have used tasks that involved a behavioral consequence. Walking on a belt moving over an electrified grid or solving a temporal food maze are two such examples. Both tasks associate drug-compensatory performance with a favorable outcome: Shock is avoided, or food is obtained. Studies of acute tolerance in humans also are typically conducted without a consideration of the consequence of performance under alcohol. Thus the extent to which this important factor influences the results of these studies is unknown. It seems that even though studies have controlled the frequency of task practice under alcohol, they may not have achieved their goal of excluding the learning that affects acute tolerance.

Our research demonstrated that learning an Rc-S* expectancy during a dose of alcohol greatly enhanced acute tolerance. This evidence indicates that acute tolerance cannot be explained *solely* by an increasing physiological adaptation to the presence of alcohol during the dose. Our findings, of course, in no way negate the possibility that such an adaption may be occurring. However, our theory predicts that the acquisition of an Rc-S* expectancy should contribute independently to enhance resistance to the effect of a dose of alcohol. One approach to demonstrating the independent effect of the Rc-S* expectancy is suggested by considering that learning effects should endure to affect subsequent behavior in the same situation. The next section describes research that examines the profile of impairment under a dose of alcohol after an Rc-S* expectancy has been learned.

## Retention Changes the Entire
## Profile of Impairment

In the studies we have just reviewed, drinkers who received the "learning" treatment should have acquired an Rc-S* expectancy by the end of the first dose. If so, then the expectancy should be retained and recur as soon as drinking begins a second time in the same situation. Because the expectancy should increase the likelihood of displaying an Rc, diminished impairment should be observed during the early *rising* BACs of the second dose. If the Rc-S* association continues to be confirmed during the second dose, the Rc-S* expectancy should become more certain. As a result, the Rc should occur more reliably, and an even greater reduction of impairment should be evident if a third dose is administered in the same situation. Given that the Rc-S* association is maintained, the occurrence of an Rc should continue to increase, and may eventually overwhelm the comparatively mild impairment initially observed during low BACs on both limbs of the alcohol curve. Therefore, performance may be *better* under alcohol than drug-free.

Theory suggests that individual differences in learning history should be detected even when the performance of all subjects is subsequently tested under identical conditions. Thus, when individuals are advised in advance that a drinking situation provides an advantageous consequence for drug-compensatory performance, those who have already learned to expect this outcome should have a head start on resisting the effect of alcohol. Therefore, when drinking occurs in a situation that presents the Rc-S* association, drinkers who have acquired a prior Rc-S* expectancy should be less impaired during the entire course of the dose than drinkers without this learning history.

These hypotheses are novel and important. They imply that a learned Rc-S* expectancy has an *enduring* effect on the *entire* profile of impairment under a dose of alcohol. When drinking occurs in a situation where the expectancy has been acquired, impairment during rising *and* declining limbs of the BAC curve should be reduced. Moreover, a well-established expectancy should have a stronger effect. Impairment at the peak BAC may be diminished, and performance during low BACs on both limbs of the curve may be better than that observed drug-free.

Tests of these predictions require the administration of repeated doses of alcohol and an examination of drug effects during rising and declining BACs of each dose. One such experiment (Vogel-Sprott, Sdao-Jarvie, & Fillmore, 1991) involved four groups of social drinkers who attended four drinking sessions. On each session, they received the same moderate dose of alcohol and performed the task ten times after drinking.

The first drinking session provided two learning groups with opportunities to associate Rc with a desirable S*. One group received the expensive form of training, a monetary S* for the display of compensatory performance under alcohol. The cheap version, an informative S* without any money, was administered to the other group. The two remainingn no-learning groups had no S* temporally contingent upon Rc. One of these groups received a cheap form of treatment in which no event was associated with performance under alcohol. The other group received an expensive variant, where money was promised for compensatory performance but no information on earnings was provided until subjects were paid at the conclusion of the experiment. The groups continued to receive their respective treatments on the next two alcohol sessions. Thus session 1 provided evidence on the effect of learning the Rc-S* expectancy during a dose of alcohol, and sessions 2 and 3 assessed the effect of continuing to confirm this expectation on subsequent drinking occasions.

By the conclusion of the third drinking session, the learning and no-learning groups could be considered to represent drinkers with and without a well-established Rc-S* expectancy. The fourth session tested the effect of this learning history. At the outset of this session, each subject was advised that money would be immediately paid for compensatory performance. Thus all drinkers knew about the Rc-S* relationship before drinking commenced, but this was new information to the no-learning group, and presumably well known by the learning group. In all other respects, the subjects were treated identically. After drinking commenced, a monetary S* was adminis-tered whenever an Rc was displayed on a trial.

The ten trials on the task during each session were scheduled at regular intervals after drinking began, and subjects' BACs were determined immediately after every trial. These BACs did not differ significantly among sessions or groups. Table 1 shows the mean (SEM) BAC during each trial, averaged over groups and sessions. The table shows the first three trials were performed while BAC was rising. A mean peak BAC of 72 mg/100 ml was obtained with the

**TABLE 1.** Mean (SEM) BAC (mg/100 ml) at Test Trial Intervals during Four Alcohol Sessions

|  | Test trials | | | | | | | | | |
|---|---|---|---|---|---|---|---|---|---|---|
|  | 1 | 2 | 3 | 4 | 5 | 6 | 7 | 8 | 9 | 10 |
| Minutes after drinking began | 20 | 40 | 60 | 70 | 80 | 90 | 100 | 110 | 120 | 130 |
| Mean BAC | 18 | 45 | 70 | 72 | 68 | 66 | 62 | 59 | 56 | 54 |
| (SEM) | 0.47 | 0.57 | 0.73 | 0.51 | 0.68 | 0.36 | 0.35 | 0.47 | 0.54 | 0.57 |

fourth trial of the session, 70 minutes after drinking commenced. The remaining six trials were performed while BAC declined.

The effect of alcohol on performance during the sessions did not differ significantly under the cheap and expensive forms of the learning treatment, and the two versions of the no-learning treatment also did not differ. Therefore, the data from the two forms of each treatment were combined, and Figure 22 shows the effect of alcohol on learning (L) and no-learning (NL) groups on each of the ten trials during drinking sessions 1, 2 and 3. The zero position on the vertical axis represents a subject's drug-free level of achievement just prior to drinking on each session. Positive changes above the drug-free baseline show impairment, and negative changes indicate improved performance under alcohol.

Figure 22 shows the first dose of alcohol yielded results consistent with those previously described in our single dose studies. On session 1, the learning and no-learning groups displayed a similar degree of impairment during the first three trials, while BAC was rising to its peak. In contrast, the learning group showed a greatly accelerated recovery from impairment during declining BACs. A comparison of the slopes of the scores on trials 5 to 10 showed the reduction in drug effect was significantly faster in the learning group.

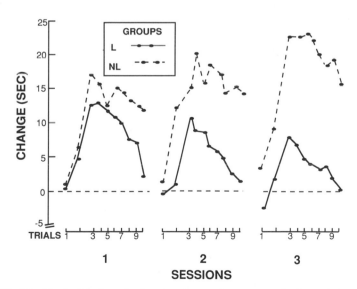

**FIGURE 22.** Alcohol-induced change in performance during rising and declining BACs during three drinking sessions providing learning (L) or no-learning (NL) treatment.

The first three trials of each session in Figure 22 test the prediction that the acquisition of an Rc-S* expectancy during one drinking occasion should be retained, and should immediately begin to diminish impairment during rising BACs when drinking starts a second time in the same situation. Furthermore, expectancy effects should strengthen if the second drinking occasion continues to confirm the Rc-S* association. Thus an even greater reduction in impairment during rising BACs should be observed under a third dose of alcohol. These results are evident in Figure 22. The learning group displayed significantly less impairment on the first three trials of session 2 than the no-learning group, and these group differences were stronger on session 3. The figure also shows the *entire* profile of impairment displayed by the learning group changed systematically over the three drinking sessions. There was a progressive reduction in impairment at the peak BAC, as well as both limbs of the blood alcohol curve. By the third session, their performance at low BACs was *better* or *equal* to their drug-free achievement. No such trends were evident in the no-learning group.

All subjects had the same number of task trials under alcohol during each session and received the same doses of alcohol under identical environmental conditions. Thus the differences between the learning and no-learning groups cannot be attributed to differences in task practice, alcohol exposure, or the expectation of drinking alcohol. Treatment effects are also not due to the sheer presence or absence of money, because cheap (no money) and expensive (money) forms of each treatment were administered. The only systematic difference between the treatments was the presence or absence of information about the advantageous consequence of drug-compensatory performance. This information was only provided by the learning treatment. Thus this factor must presumably be responsible for the findings. In theory, such information permits the acquisition of an Rc-S* expectancy. Repetitions of an Rc-S* association in a drinking situation permits the acquisition of a more certain response–outcome expectancy that increases drug-compensatory performance. The learned expectancy is retained, and thus its influence can operate immediately whenever drinking recurs in the same situation.

The learning group presumably had many opportunities to acquire an Rc-S* expectancy during the first three drinking sessions, whereas the no-learning group had no such opportunity. Session 4 tested the effect of these different learning histories in a drinking situation that provided both groups with a monetary S* for the display of drug-compensatory performance. These results are pre-

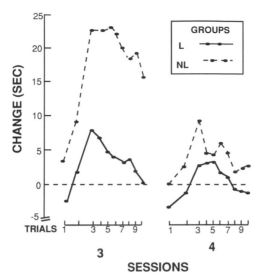

**FIGURE 23.** The effect of a history of learning (L) or no-learning (NL) training on performance under alcohol on session 4. Session 3 is included for comparison.

sented in Figure 23, and for comparison the figure also includes session 3. Significant learning history effects were demonstrated on session 4, even though all subjects were advised of the Rc-S* association prior to drinking on this session. The learning group, with a previously acquired expectancy, displayed less impairment during rising, peak, and declining BACs.

A comparison of the performance of subjects in the learning group on sessions 3 and 4 also showed that continuing confirmation of the Rc-S* association further strengthened resistance to impairment. On session 4, their performance at both ends of the BAC curve had become *better* under alcohol than drug-free. The effect of introducing the Rc-S* association to subjects who had not had a previous opportunity to relate these two events is shown by comparing the performance of the no-learning group on sessions 3 and 4. This group had no S* associated with Rc until the fourth dose. Figure 23 shows the preparatory instructions about the Rc-S* relationship, and its confirmation during trials on session 4 greatly diminished the impairment of the no-learning group. However, without the benefit of a prior learned Rc-S* expectancy, the group was still more impaired under the fourth dose than was the learning group.

## Summary

The evidence reviewed in this chapter leads to the following conclusions:

1. An Rc-S* expectancy acquired during a single drinking occasion can enhance acute tolerance (i.e., hasten recovery during declining BACs).

2. An acquired expectancy enhances resistance to the effect of both rising *and* declining BACs on subsequent drinking occasions in a similar situation.

3. When the expectancy is well established, it provides a drinker with a head start on diminishing the impairing effect of a dose, and alters the entire profile of behavior during all phases of the BAC curve. Impairment is diminished overall, and drug effects may be reversed so that *improved* performance is displayed at low BACs on both limbs of the blood alcohol curve.

4. A learned Rc-S* expectancy has an enduring effect on the response to a dose of alcohol. Drinkers with and without a prior learned expectancy display a different profile of impairment, even when they all know in advance that a drinking situation will provide an advantageous consequence for drug-compensatory performance.

Research interest in acute tolerance languished for decades while investigators attempted to determine that acute alcohol tolerance was not simply an artifact of task practice. That evidence has now been received, and contemporary research interest has favored the pursuit of the "pure" phenomenon of acute tolerance, uncontaminated by task practice under alcohol.

Investigations of acute tolerance in humans have invested heavily in the assumption that the phenomenon can be examined separately from learning by controlling the amount of task practice under alcohol. However, our research suggests that task practice is important only insofar as it provides an opportunity to learn the consequences of behavior under alcohol. The influential learning factor determining a drinker's tolerance to alcohol is the expected relationship between drug-compensatory performance (Rc) and an advantageous outcome (S*). This learned Rc-S* expectancy can have a great impact on acute tolerance. Acquiring information about the Rc-S* association during a single dose can raise the BAC threshold for recovery from alcohol effects and greatly abbreviate the duration of impairment. In addition, when an individual has acquired an Rc-S* expectancy pertinent to a situation in which drinking occurs again, the profile of behavioral effects over the entire blood alcohol curve is dramatically altered. Impairment is greatly reduced during all phases under the dose, and impairment may be reversed to show improved performance at each end of the BAC curve. The effect of an Rc-S* expectancy is robust and powerful. When a dose of alcohol is administered to drinkers with and without this prior learned expectancy, the difference in their response is as large as that observed between light and very heavy drinkers (Goldberg, 1943).

The effect of learning an Rc-S* association on reducing impairment under a dose of alcohol is consistent with the results in previous chapters that showed this learning had a similar effect on tolerance to repeated doses. In both cases, a diminished responsiveness to alcohol effects occurred when drinkers had information about the association between drug-compensatory performance and a desirable consequence. These findings implicate the Rc-S* expectancy as a common factor enhancing resistance to the effect of both single *and* repeated doses of alcohol.

Many investigators have speculated that acute and chronic tolerance may be influenced by some similar factors, but there has been no agreement on the factors that may be responsible (e.g., Beirness & Vogel-Sprott, 1984b; Greizerstein & Smith, 1973; Goldberg, 1943; Maynert & Klingman, 1960; Tabakoff, Ritzman, Raju, & Deitrich, 1980; Vogel-Sprott, 1979). Adaptation induced by drug exposure has been a frequent suspect. Yet the effect of the expectancy factor in our research cannot be explained by exposure to alcohol, because drug doses were identical in groups who differed markedly in tolerance to repeated doses, and impairment under a single dose. The amount of task practice under alcohol is often thought to introduce learning that affects tolerance. Yet the results of our research are not attributable to task practice per se, because groups were also equated on this factor. When a drinker has learned to expect a desirable outcome for compensating for a given behavioral effect of alcohol, this learning can operate to diminish the drug effect. Its effects act swiftly. Even as the expectancy is being acquired, it can accelerate recovery from a dose of alcohol. The expectancy is also retained. When drinking recurs in a situation where the expectancy has been acquired, the effect of alcohol is diminished during all phases of the blood alcohol curve.

The conclusion that learned Rc-S* expectancies are an important determinant of the acute and chronic tolerance displayed by social drinkers has several theoretical and practical ramifications. It carries some important implications for understanding the risk of alcohol abuse and its treatment. This conclusion is also clearly at variance with the customary view of alcohol tolerance and dependence as a single process. The results of our research program raise many questions that will require investigation. In addition, the findings of our experiments have some potential application to social settings. Here they lead to some rather provocative notions concerning alcohol-related accidents and the responsibility for drunken comportment in society. These topics are discussed in the next chapters.

# VI

IMPLICATIONS
AND
APPLICATIONS

# 9

## Theory and Research

$C$hapter 4 presented a theoretical analysis of events that could affect expectancies in a drinking situation. The theory identified a particular response–outcome expectancy (Rc-S*) as an important determinant of social drinkers' behavioral tolerance to alcohol, and our research provided considerable support for this hypothesis. It seems that the theoretical model has promising predictive potential. This chapter discusses some additional hypotheses and implications for research.

### Predicting Behavioral Tolerance

The discussion requires reference to our theoretical model. It was presented in Figure 3B of Chapter 4 as:

| S | ⟶ | Sd* | ⟶ | Rc | ⟶ | S* |
|---|---|-----|---|----|---|-----|
| stimulus cues predicting drug | | drug stimulus | | compensatory response | | desirable outcome |

The S and the Sd* symbolize the distinctive environmental events (S) associated with the administration of a drug (Sd*). Learning the S-Sd* relationship provides a stimulus–outcome expectancy: Alcohol is expected in this situation, and this sets the stage for a drinking occasion. An R by itself stands for any behavioral response that may occur under alcohol. For any given activity, a drug-like (Rd) or a drug-opposite response (Rc) may be displayed. Drug-like responses are identified as symptoms of alcohol intoxication. Symptoms of tolerance are identified by drug-opposite responses that serve to compensate for the drug effects. Of course, the exact nature of the symptoms depends upon the activity examined. For example, an assessment of car driving could reveal impaired or improved reaction time, but not the presence or absence of slurred speech.In theory, the consequences of displaying intoxication or tolerance depend upon the particular activity and the drinking situation. Information about a reliable R-S* association provides a drinker with a response–outcome expectancy that is specific to the activity and the situation. The expectancy serves an adaptive function, allowing behavior to be modified to attain the most desirable outcome. From this perspective, the expression of behavioral symptoms in a drinking situation is flexible and adjusts to the environmental conditions. If intoxication has a more desirable consequence than tolerance, drug-like symptoms of intoxication should be displayed. If tolerance yields a more desirable consequence, a drug-compensatory response will be exhibited. Our experiments demonstrated this principle by considering one activity, psychomotor performance, and the consequence of compensating for one symptom, impairment. But the theoretical explanation is general, and it makes the same prediction concerning the presence or absence of tolerance in any other activity that may occur during a drinking occasion.

The theory predicts that a drinker could display alcohol tolerance in the performance of a given activity in one situation, and no tolerance when the same activity is performed on another drinking occasion. This should be observed whenever a desirable consequence for drug-compensatory performance of an activity is present in one situation and absent in another. For example, a drinker who must make a banquet address is likely to expect drug-tolerant speech to yield a much more desirable consequence than slurred diction. Tolerance should be displayed under these conditions, and therefore symptoms of intoxication in speech may not be evident. On the other hand, the drinker's speech may be slurred after consuming the same amount of alcohol at a party among close friends, because no special advantage accrues for drug-tolerant speech. The research on the extinction of tolerance, discussed in Chapter 6, provides another example. Here the tolerance acquired when drug-compensatory performance was associated with a favorable consequence was extinguished on subsequent drinking occasions that withheld this expected outcome. The monetary consequence used in this research on extinction could convey information about drug-compensatory performance as well as an incentive to display this behavior. Hence the extinction of tolerance when the monetary consequence was withheld might be due to the removal of the expected information, or the incentive, or both. Other research is required to separate the effect of withdrawing information from the effect of withdrawing an incentive.

In theory, the expected consequence of a given activity determines whether a drinker will display intoxication or tolerance. Because social drinkers perform many different tasks during a single drinking occasion, it would be no surprise if a drinker displayed symptoms of intoxication in some activity, and tolerance in another. This was observed incidentally in our experiments, where psychomotor performance was the only activity that had any consequence. Subjects displayed symptoms of intoxication in other behavior. They typically became more talkative after drinking. Loud exuberant laughter increased, speech was slurred, and ataxia was displayed. As a result, the experimenter often needed to assist subjects back to the laboratory to perform the task. Even so, those drinkers who expected a desirable consequence for compensating for psychomotor impairment still often displayed complete tolerance in their performance of the task. These observations are consistent with our learning analysis, but their verification remains to be determined.

There are also stories of drinkers exhibiting gross intoxication who have no difficulty whatever in performing the precise coordinated eye–hand maneuvers required to fit door and ignition keys in car locks. This simultaneous display of intoxication and tolerance also may be attributed to the different expected consequences of these activities. The drug-tolerant performance required to enter and start a car is more desirable than remaining impaired but stranded. In this situation there is no comparable gain for compensating for other symptoms, such as slurred speech or ataxia. Unless, of course, the individual is stopped by the police during the drive home. The presence of a police officer changes the situation. Now the expected consequences of displaying tolerance to *all* symptoms of intoxication are more desirable. Under such circumstances, evidence of intoxication should be much more difficult to obtain. This hypothesis also remains to be tested.

Such a prediction is particularly interesting because drinkers likely encounter many situations in which the display of tolerance to all symptoms of intoxication is advantageous. This was illustrated by the anecdote in Chapter 2 that described the remarkable display of tolerance by impaired drivers undergoing clinical assessments by police physicians. Other data also suggest that impairment in such situations is extremely difficult to detect. In the past, several countries required all drivers accused of impaired driving to be examined by a medical officer. A review of the results (National Safety Council, 1968) showed that physicians could only identify half the drivers with BACs of 100 mg/100 ml or higher as impaired. When drivers were stopped on city streets, highly trained interviewers correctly identified only 45% of the drivers that had BACs at or over 100 mg/100 ml (Zusman & Huber, 1979). Police officers interviewing motorists at checkpoints also have great difficulty in detecting symptoms of intoxication. Vingilis, Adlaf, and Chung (1982) found that they failed to identify 95% of the drivers who had BACs of 80 mg/100 ml and higher. Jones and Lund (1986) found police failed to identify 55% of drivers with BACs over 100 mg/100 ml. When breath tests were obtained on all drivers who *passed* police scrutiny at a sobriety checkpoint, it was found that only 33% of drivers with BACs at or over 100 mg/100 ml were identified (Worden, Flynn, Merrill, Waller, & Haugh, 1989).

Langenbucher and Nathan (1983) have reported that symptoms of intoxication in social drinkers and alcoholics are extremely difficult to detect in a variety of circumstances. A retrospective analysis of these situations suggests that they are ones where symptoms of intoxication are likely to be socially unacceptable and tolerance is advantageous. In a similar vein, Sobell, Sobell, and VanderSpek (1979) concluded that trained observers could not make valid estimates of the sobriety of individuals when they were assessed during follow-up or admission to alcoholism treatment facilities.

It is obvious that the display of behavioral tolerance when it is advantageous must be limited to conditions where a drinker's BAC has not risen to a level that induces stupor or coma. But there is no evidence yet to indicate whether the ability to compensate for the symptoms of intoxication progressively diminishes as BAC becomes higher, or whether tolerance is well maintained until some critical high BAC is reached and a drinker collapses. This latter possibility is implied in many anecdotes about individuals who drink a large amount of alcohol with no apparent effects, and only suddenly display gross intoxication.

A number of studies have examined the drinking behavior of alcoholics under experimental conditions (Mello & Mendelson, 1965, 1970; Mendelson & Mello, 1966; Mendelson, Stein, & Mello, 1965; Nathan, Lowenstein, Solomon, & Rossi, 1970; Nathan & O'Brien, 1971; Nathan, O'Brien, & Lowenstein, 1971). Some of these studies also suggest that drinkers having extraordinarily high BACs can still display behavioral tolerance when it is advantageous (Mello &

Mendelson, 1965; Mendelson & Mello, 1966; Nathan, Titler, Lowenstein, Solomon, & Rossi, 1970). This research examined the drinking patterns of male alcohol abusers who performed operant tasks for points that could be exchanged for alcohol. Mello and Mendelson found that BACs in excess of 250 mg/100 ml rarely produced any symptoms of intoxication, and subjects performed the tasks with good accuracy. In contrast, the studies by Nathan and his colleagues found that BACs above 200 mg/100 ml resulted in gross impairment and ataxia. Nathan et al. (1970) suggested that the inconsistent observation of symptoms of intoxication in the two sets of studies may be due to the different environmental settings in which the experiments were conducted. Our analysis would go one step further to identify the source of the discrepancy with the different consequences of behavior in the two drinking environments.

The subjects in Nathan's experiments could accumulate points during nondrinking periods to spend on subsequent drinking days. This offered subjects the option of not working on the task during drinking periods. As a result, tolerance to the impairing effects of alcohol had no particular advantage. Symptoms of intoxication could be displayed without penalizing the accrual of alcohol. In contrast, the studies of Mello and Mendelson required subjects to perform the task for points *while* drinking. Therefore, they could not drink unless they compensated for the drug effect and performed the task successfully. In addition, Nathan's subjects resided in a separate facility, but drinkers in Mello and Mendelson's studies were in a general psychiatric ward amid a group of sober, mostly female patients. Their attitude to an intoxicated male is a matter of conjecture, but it seems likely that drinkers in such a ward would find the display of tolerance to be advantageous.

## Expectancy and Capability

We have found that social drinkers' Rc-S* expectancies provided a very reliable guide to the behavioral tolerance they displayed. It is reasonable to suppose that these expectancies could enhance tolerance only if a drinker's behavioral repertoire included a compensatory response. Expecting a favorable outcome for drug-compensatory performance is unlikely to affect tolerance when a drinker does not know how to adjust behavior to compensate for the drug effect. Our research did not examine this possibility. Our studies were designed to demonstrate that drug exposure per se was not sufficient to guarantee a compensatory reaction, and that tolerance was enhanced by mental or overt repetitions of an Rc-S* association. Such practice could strengthen an Rc-S* expectancy. However, it also might simultaneously permit the acquisition of a new behavioral strategy to compensate for the effect of alcohol on task performance.

Drinkers may not need to learn how to compensate for alcohol effects if tasks are very simple. In such cases, an Rc-S* expectancy may be sufficient to enhance tolerance. However, as tasks become more demanding and complex, it may be necessary to learn some new task-specific coping strategies to compensate for the effect of alcohol. If so, then this learning may be required before tolerance can be activated by an Rc-S* expectancy. There are many possible sources of learning about a compensatory behavioral strategy. Performance under drug that rewards compensatory performance may be one example: *drug-free* training of a complex task under conditions that mimic alcohol effects may be another. This latter possibility is particularly interesting in view of the evidence that the effect of the first administration of a drug to an animal can be influenced by its prior drug-free experiences (Barrett et al., 1989). The reasons for these effects are not known, but one possibility is that the drug-free history of performance results in a learned response that increases the capability to display tolerance. If a priori drug-free training could provide a drinker with a behavioral strategy to compensate for alcohol, tolerance could be more readily expressed on the first drinking occasion that provides an advantageous outcome for compensating. Some current research in our laboratory provides promising support for this speculation (Zinatelli, 1992).

## Individual Differences

Our research has accumulated considerable evidence showing that social drinkers display a remarkable degree of alcohol tolerance when they expect an advantageous consequence (S*) for compensatory performance (Rc). The presence of an Rc-S* association on a single drinking occasion greatly enhanced social drinkers' resistance to the behavioral effect of the alcohol. In addition, consistent and enduring differences in tolerance were observed among drinkers with or without a prior opportunity to acquire an Rc-S* expectancy. Although our research examined the effect of alcohol on the performance of complex psychomotor tasks, the results may be generally applicable to other tasks and activities performed by humans during drinking occasions. This possibility remains to be investigated, because the

Rc-S* association in drinking situations has not previously been identified as an important determinant of the behavioral effect of alcohol.

If the results of our research can be demonstrated to generalize to other activities, they would raise important questions about the interpretation of the findings in experiments that measure individual differences in the behavioral effect of a dose of alcohol. Many experiments have administered a challenge dose of alcohol to investigate the response of different groups of individuals that may be at risk for alcoholism. Two such examples are persons with either a positive or a negative family history of alcoholism (see, e.g., Newlin & Thomson, 1990), or light versus very heavy drinkers (see, e.g., Goldberg, 1943). These studies typically administer a single dose of alcohol to all groups of subjects and test the behavioral effects under identical conditions. When such experiments find certain groups show more or less acute tolerance or impairment under a dose of alcohol, the result is attributed to the effect of the alcohol-related characteristic that distinguished the groups. However, such characteristics also may have provided groups with different learned Rc-S* expectancies that could greatly influence their response to alcohol. Humans enter experiments with rich and varied histories of drinking experiences that could create individual differences in the expected consequences of compensating for a given behavioral effect of alcohol. Some research indicates that alcohol expectancies differ among individuals, and these expectancies may be influenced by the setting (Sher, 1985).

An individual's drinking customs, as well as family and peer group attitudes toward drinking, are likely sources of individual differences in expectations about what particular behavior under alcohol has what consequence. These expectancies may provide important guidance, allowing a drinker to anticipate what particular behavior is most desirable in a specific social context. Some drinkers may have well-established Rc-S* expectancies that are pertinent to the experimental situation, and others may have none. Thus, when different groups of drinkers with different alcohol-related characterisitics are compared, the interpretation of the results of single-dose studies is equivocal. Are differences in the response to alcohol due to group differences in prior learned Rc-S* expectancies, or the alcohol-related characteristic that defined the group, or both?

## Predicting Placebo Responses to Alcohol

Previous chapters reviewed many studies showing that alcohol tolerance is increased by the expectation of an advantageous outcome

(S*) for a response (Rc) that compensates for the drug effect. In these experiments, alcohol impaired performance by slowing reactions on psychomotor tasks. Thus the compensatory response, Rc, opposite in direction to the influence of the drug, should increase the speed of reactions on the task. Because a dose of a drug is thought to exert a constant effect, the development of tolerance presumably is due to strengthening Rc. Our research was in line with this view and demonstrated that drinkers with an opportunity to acquire an Rc-S* expectancy displayed greater behavioral tolerance to alcohol than those without this expectancy training. Additional and more direct confirmation of the expectancy prediction was provided by experiments that substituted a placebo for alcohol on a drinking session after tolerance was established. The placebo consistently revealed a drug-opposite response (Rc) whose strength could be predicted by the degree of tolerance previously displayed: Drinkers with an acquired Rc-S* expectancy showed a stronger Rc.

There is a very large literature on the social drinker's responses to placebo drinks. Reviews of this work concur in the conclusion that placebo responses are absent in motor skill tasks (Hull & Bond, 1986; Marlatt & Rohsenow, 1980; Rohsenow & Marlatt, 1981). No drug-like (Rd) or drug-opposite (Rc) reactions to placebo appear to be obtained in psychomotor behavior. Yet our placebo research used motor skill tasks and consistently demonstrated the occurrence of Rc. Why other placebo experiments have failed to obtain any reliable effects in motor behavior and our studies have succeeded is an interesting puzzle. Our theoretical analysis offers an explanation.

Most studies testing placebo responses to alcohol employ a single drinking session. Many studies have used a balanced placebo design in which four groups of subjects receive a drink. Two receive alcohol, and two receive a placebo. Within each beverage condition, one group is told that the drink is alcohol, the other is told that the drink is a placebo, usually tonic water. Comparisons among the four groups permit the effect of expecting alcohol to be distinguished from the pharmacological effect of the drug. These studies manipulate the expectation of receiving alcohol by telling subjects the drink is alcoholic and presenting salient cues for alcohol, such as familiar alcohol scents and bottles, when the placebo drink is served. Our presentation of the placebo is similar, and in this respect our studies may be comparable. In terms of our theory, this expectancy is identified as S-Sd* and is considered a prerequisite for the occurrence of a placebo reaction. There has been some debate over whether the cues used in balanced placebo design experiments lead drinkers to believe they have received alcohol (Collins & Searles, 1988; Knight,

Barbaree, & Boland, 1986). However, the creation of this expectancy seems likely to be adequate because it usually results in either drug-like or drug-opposite placebo reactions in social and affective behaviors (Hull & Bond, 1986; Marlatt & Rohsenow, 1980). The more interesting question is why an S-Sd* expectancy evokes no placebo reaction in psychomotor behavior in single drinking session experiments, whereas our studies have been so successful in obtaining a drug-opposite placebo response.

From our perspective, tolerance and the reaction to a placebo both depend upon more than the expectation of drinking alcohol. Our theory identified four important events, S, Sd*, R, and S*, that affect behavior in a drinking situation. These events provide information not only about receiving alcohol, but also about the effect of the drug on a particular activity, and the consequence of displaying the effect in a drinking situation. Unlike single-session placebo studies, our experiments involved a number of drinking sessions that provided some groups of subjects with an opportunity to acquire this information *prior* to a placebo test. Thus, although alcohol was expected when the placebo was received, a drug-opposite response was most evident in groups who had learned to expect a desirable consequence for compensating. When an individual believes alcohol has been consumed, it may be that additional expectancies about the type of response and its consequence determine whether a placebo response will be reliably observed, and whether it will be drug-like (Rd) or drug-opposite (Rc) (Vogel-Sprott & Fillmore, 1991).

Although psychomotor performance may reveal either drug-like or drug-opposite responses to a placebo, our experiments observed only a drug-opposite reaction. This may be attributed to the experimental treatment that preceded our placebo test. Because of our interest in tolerance, repeated doses of alcohol were administered on drinking occasions that provided a reliable association between drug-compensatory performance (Rc) and an advantageous outcome (S*). This training permitted the acquisition of information leading to the expectation that compensatory performance could be displayed, and that it had the most favorable consequence. Thus this set of expectancies may explain why a drug-opposite placebo response was subsequently displayed when drinkers thought that they had received alcohol.

This analysis suggests that when drinkers believe they have consumed alcohol, a reliable placebo reaction should be obtainable in psychomotor or other types of activities, *provided that* the drinkers also have similar expectancies concerning the type of reaction to alcohol and its consequence. A drug-opposite placebo response should be displayed by drinkers who expect that they can compensate for the drug effect, and that the consequence of displaying compensation is more favorable than that of displaying intoxication. A drug-like placebo response should be observed when drinkers expect that the display of symptoms of intoxication have a more advantageous consequence or no penalizing consequence. Some recent research on placebo responses to caffeine has provided promising support for these predictions (Fillmore, 1990; Fillmore & Vogel-Sprott, 1992).

From this perspective, the failure of single drinking session experiments to observe any reliable placebo response in psychomotor behavior would be attributed to the failure of drinkers to share a common set of expectations concerning the type of response to be made to alcohol and the consequence of the response in a given drinking situation. This interpretation also implies that studies using a balanced placebo design have successfully detected placebo reactions in social behavior because subjects entering the experiment have already acquired the same requisite set of expectancies concerning this behavior under alcohol and its outcome. Prior cultural and social experiences may train many expectations concerning the type of symptoms, and the consequences of exhibiting these symptoms in particular drinking situations. It is interesting to note that this theoretical explanation for the occurrence of placebo responses is similar in many respects to other speculations concerning the reason that placebo effects regularly occur only in social behavior (Marlatt & Rohsenow, 1980; Rohsenow & Marlatt, 1981).

## Summary

Research described in previous chapters demonstrated that the consequence of a behavior in a drinking situation, and the learned expectation of the consequence, predicted the degree of tolerance a drinker displayed. Moreover, these results were obtained when drinkers' alcohol consumption was identical. Thus it appears that the amount of alcohol used by social drinkers cannot predict the amount of behavioral tolerance they display to the drug. Such a conclusion is consistent with our theory. From our perspective, the important factor is a drinker's learning history concerning the consequences of behavior under alcohol. The particular learning history that characterizes a drinker, together with the consequences in a drinking situation, predict the behavioral tolerance displayed. The implications of this conclusion, and hypotheses for future research, were discussed in the present chapter.

The theoretical explanation for the variability in the alcohol tolerance displayed by a social drinker was illustrated by analyzing three examples:

1. A drinker displays drug-tolerant performance of a task in one setting, and no tolerance when the same task is performed in a different drinking situation.
2. Alternating symptoms of intoxication and tolerance are observed in a drinker's performance of the same activity during a single drinking occasion.
3. A drinker performs different tasks in a drinking situation and displays tolerance in some, but none in others.

The tolerance-enhancing effect of expecting an advantageous consequence for compensating was considered to require that a drinker's behavioral repertoire includes a response strategy for compensating for alcohol effects on performance. The strategy presumably had to be available before the expectancy could exert an influence. It was suggested this may be especially relevant to extremely complex tasks. Whereas it seemed likely that such a strategy might be learned by performing under alcohol, it was suggested that such learning also may occur in drug-free situations that include disrupting stimuli that have effects similar to those of alcohol.

The evidence for an enduring influence of learned expectations on a drinker's alcohol tolerance prompted some questions concerning the appropriateness of assessing individual differences by administering a single challenge dose of alcohol. Many such experiments compare drinkers who differ on some characteristic that may indicate a risk of alcohol abuse. When differences are observed, they are attributed to the characteristic that distinguished the groups. However, the groups are also likely to come to an experiment with very different drinking experiences that could provide very different learning histories with respect to the expected consequences of compensating for the effect of alcohol. Thus it seemed that the interpretation of the individual differences in single dose studies could be perplexing.

The failure of other research to obtain any reliable placebo response to alcohol in psychomotor behavior was discussed. The response–outcome expectancy theory suggested that the failure may be attributable to a failure to control or train important expectancies that affect the occurrences of a placebo response. In addition, the analysis suggested that the acquisition of specific response–outcome expectancies could explain and predict drug-like and drug-opposite responses to a placebo dose of alcohol.

# 10

## Transition from Social to Abusive Drinking

Our research identified some neglected factors that affect the alcohol tolerance of social drinkers. The evidence indicated that their behavioral tolerance resembled adaptive learning and may be an extremely common, normal phenomenon. These findings have implications for understanding the role their behavioral tolerance may play in promoting alcohol abuse. The view suggested by our research is discussed in this chapter. Differences between this perspective and traditionally accepted notions of tolerance, and the risk of escalating alcohol consumption, also are discussed.

### Behavioral Tolerance and Physical Dependence

Although it is only possible to speculate about the nature of the adaptive mechanism underlying the tolerance, our evidence on social drinkers implies that the mechanism must involve perceptual and cognitive processes. This conclusion is clearly at odds with the traditional view of tolerance as an involuntary adaptive reaction that restores biological homeostasis in the presence of alcohol. Our experimental treatments caused social drinkers to display a remarkable degree of tolerance with no vestige of withdrawal distress that could be considered to indicate physical dependence. This evidence cannot be reconciled with the opinion "that alcohol tolerance and physical dependence are closely related phenomena, which develop essentially in parallel in man" (Kalant, 1975, p. 5).

Tolerance and physical dependence usually have been considered to be two sides of the same coin. Although the literature on alcohol reports that exceptional tolerance may be displayed by individuals who are not physically dependent upon alcohol (Jellinek, 1960), tolerance and dependence are customarily attributed to a single adaptive mechanism. Under drug, this reaction restores homeostasis, so tolerance is observed. When the drug is withheld, the reaction is observed as withdrawal distress. The assumption of a common mechanism underlying tolerance and physical dependence implies that the same process *initiates* tolerance and *sustains* it during all stages of alcohol use. In contrast, our research implies that the processes accounting for tolerance during early stages of alcohol use differ from mechanisms that may sustain tolerance after dependence is established. It seems that the tolerance developed by social drinkers during early stages of alcohol use may depend importantly, and possibly chiefly, upon learning processes.

The notion that one mechanism accounts for *all* instances of alcohol tolerance has given rise to polarized stands. Some have argued that the mechanism is entirely learning (e.g., Wenger et al., 1981), whereas others hold the process to be an involuntary physiological adaptation to the action of the drug (e.g., LeBlanc et al., 1973). But each camp encounters data that it cannot explain. Wolgin (1989) and Kalant (1987) have noted that exceptions to each position are evident when the results of prolonged high alcohol doses are contrasted with shorter low-dose exposures. For example, prolonged exposure of animals to alcohol vapor in a closed chamber will produce alcohol tolerance and withdrawal symptoms indicating physical dependence (Goldstein, 1972). This massive respiratory exposure to alcohol is unlike any exposure humans are likely to encounter. This procedure appears to exclude any opportunity for learned responses under the drug, and cannot be explained if tolerance is solely dependent upon learning processes. On the other hand, an account of tolerance solely in terms of physiological adaptation to the drug cannot explain why environmental events that influence learning can alter the tolerance of subjects who receive the same doses of alcohol. One possibility is that learning and physiological adaptation can each produce tolerance, but the balance of their influence shifts from one to the other as the degree and intensity of drug exposure increases. The influence of learning may diminish as continuing exposure to high doses gives rise to physical dependence. At this later stage, tolerance may be determined primarily by some as yet unidentified involuntary physiological adaptation to the pharmacological action of the drug.

## Early and Late Stages of Tolerance

Tolerance after continuous exposure to alcohol vapor in a closed chamber could be considered as a "late " stage example because physical dependence was also obtained. With the occurrence of physical dependence, biological adaptation to the pharmacological action of the drug may greatly determine the display of tolerance. The effect of learning variables on alcohol tolerance is usually demonstrated in experiments that administer moderate doses and comparatively slight exposure—four or five repetitions of the dose. These conditions seem to qualify as an "early" stage of drug exposure and bear a resemblance to the manner in which social drinkers use alcohol. From our perspective, learning processes should play the important role in determining tolerance *prior* to the development of physical dependence.

Kalant (1987) has commented on the difficulties of attributing all instances of tolerance to a single process. He left open the possibility that there may be more than one mechanism of tolerance but argued for a parsimonious assumption. He suggested that the stimulus to the development of tolerance is not the presence of the drug per se, or its direct molecular interaction with a specific receptor. Rather, the stimulus is the functional impairment produced by the drug. "Neurons or synapses, in an altered state associated with functional activity, are more sensitive to the effects of ethanol and other drugs and therefore experience a greater stimulus to adapt to these effects" (Kalant, 1987, p. 13). In essence, this proposal retains a single physiological adaptive mechanism by assuming that this process accelerates when neurons or synapses are in an altered state associated with functional activity. The assumption that behavior under alcohol hastens, but does not fundamentally alter, the physiological process of adaptation is called "behaviorally augmented" tolerance (LeBlanc et al., 1973, 1975b).

However, behaviorally augmented tolerance does not explain our evidence on social drinkers, because they were equated in terms of either physical or mental activity under alcohol. Their treatment differed only with respect to the consequence (S*) of the activity. The differences in tolerance resulting from these treatments contradict the assumption that an increase in functional demands enhances tolerance by stimulating biological adaptation to alcohol.

It seems unlikely that alcohol tolerance is a stable global physiological state of resistance to a drug. The determinants of social drinkers' tolerance appear to be better explained by the relationships between drug effects, responses, and consequences that have been learned. Of course, learning has biological ramifications that may alter synapses and neurons, so behavioral tolerance is still ultimately based upon biological events. Given that learned associations between alcohol-related events predict alcohol tolerance, these influences are most likely to be evident at low doses of alcohol that do not create stupor or massive disruption of the central nervous system. Under high doses, the opportunity to learn, or to express what has been learned, may not have detectable effects on tolerance.

In the absence of massive doses of alcohol, tolerance should be governed by learned expectancies specific to activities and consequences in a given situation. This led to our proposal that a drinker could simultaneously display tolerance in one activity and none in another. Other research also shows that animals under moderate doses of alcohol will only display tolerance to some effects of the dose (Le, Khanna, & Kalant, 1984).

The evidence on social drinkers suggested that behavioral symptoms of intoxication or tolerance are determined by the expected consequence of the behavior under alcohol. One important implication of this conclusion is that social drinkers are not hapless victims of the effects of alcohol. As far as behavior is concerned, it is adaptive and guided by a drinker's expectation of the sort of response that yields the most favorable outcome in the situation. Further, these expectancies may be learned without repeated overt performance under alcohol. Mentally rehearsing a response and its consequence under alcohol was very effective in promoting a high degree of behavioral tolerance. The tolerance-inducing effect of mental rehearsal is a new finding that has not previously been demonstrated. Traditional theories of drug tolerance might consider the results remarkable, but outside this framework the findings would be no surprise. Cognitive behavioral therapy has long recognized the adaptive benefits of mentally rehearsing coping responses in the presence of real or imaginary disrupting stimuli (Meichenbaum, 1977).

The results of mental rehearsal raise the possibility that social drinkers may glean response–outcome information about behavior under alcohol from many sources. Social models are one possible example. Individuals may observe other drinkers' behavior and accrued consequences. Explicit verbal instructions about particular response–outcome contingencies, as well as cultural and social customs all may provide information about the sorts of behavior and resulting consequences that occur after drinking. Drinkers who receive response–outcome information from an identical source should display similar behavior after drinking. Our experiments demonstrated this effect in psychomotor performance, but the effect may be applicable to behavior in general. This remains to be tested. Conclusions that are consistent with our hypothesis have been expressed in reviews of aggression and crimes of violence in relationship to alcohol. For example, Pernanen (1976) pointed out that the evidence relating drinking to crimes of violence is only correlational, and statistical correlation does not reveal causation: The drinking and the aggression may result from some other factor. Pernanen's assessment of the evidence led him to conclude that the cause may lie in a drinker's membership in a subculture where "violent behavior is necessary and condoned in order to function" (Pernanen, 1976, p. 438). In other words, within some groups of drinkers, violent, aggressive behavior under alcohol is adaptive, and guided by the expectation that this behavior yields the most desirable consequence.

Our research led to the conclusion that a subject should acquire tolerance in a situation where (1) some response can oppose a symptom of alcohol intoxication, (2) a reliable consequence can be associated with the compensatory response, and (3) the consequence of compensating is more favorable than exhibiting intoxication. The generality of the conclusion remains to be determined, but some animal research suggests it may apply to the development of tolerance to other effects of alcohol. Le, Kalant, and Khanna (1986) found that the development of tolerance to the hypothermic effect of alcohol in rats depended upon whether the drug was administered in a hot or cold room. Tolerance was displayed only when the drug administrations occurred in a cold room, where a compensatory hyperthermic response was advantageous.

More recent experiments also point to learning as a separate adaptive mechanism in tolerance. Le, Kalant, and Khanna (1989) administered high doses of alcohol (2 or 4 g/kg for 33–35 days) to different groups of rats that received or did not receive intoxicated task practice (walking on a moving belt over an electrified grid). Subsequent tests of tolerance showed the experience of intoxicated task practice increased behavioral tolerance and its retention. In contrast, tolerance to the hypothermic and hypnotic effects of alcohol only increased as a function of the dosage administered to the rats during the chronic treatment period. Other research with rats has also distinguished a learned component in tolerance to alcohol (MacKenzie-Taylor & Rech, 1991). In this study, high doses of alcohol (2.0–2.7 g/kg) were administered intermittently or chronically to groups of animals, and the opportunity to experience the hypo-thermic effect of alcohol was manipulated under each treatment regimen. A learning effect was indicated by showing that the expe-rienced groups were more tolerant to the hypothermic effect of alcohol than the inexperienced groups. Evidence of cellular adaption was obtained from the inexperienced groups, where tolerance was evident following chronic, but not intermittent, alcohol treatment.

## Tolerance to Pleasant Outcomes

Experimenters should be able to enhance tolerance to a variety of behavioral effects of alcohol. All that is required is some ingenuity in devising a situation where a subject has a response to compensate for the drug effect, and the compensatory response can be associated with the most favorable outcome. In contrast to observable behavior, mood and emotional responses have some features that may make the creation of such a tolerance-enhancing situation difficult, if not impossible, to devise. Although mood and emotions are clearly perceptible to a drinker, their occurrence cannot be reliably deter-mined by an observer. Thus the association between drug-induced feelings and some environmental consequence cannot be controlled by an experimenter. The desirable consequence of feelings seems primarily, if not totally, a matter of private judgment. If the affective states induced by alcohol are perceived to be unpleasant, the use of the drug is likely to cease and there is no need to develop a drug-compensatory response. However, if the consequences are deemed desirable, alcohol may be readministered. Each administra-tion provides an opportunity to associate alcohol with altered feelings that have desirable consequences. In this situation, the drug-induced symptom has a more favorable outcome. There appears to be no means of altering this association because the consequence is self-administered on the basis of internal feeling states. From a drinker's viewpoint, there is no payoff for becoming tolerant to drug effects that yield pleasurable consequences. In theory, this is the very circumstance in which tolerance is most unlikely to develop.

Research on alcohol and other drugs has led some investigators to consider that tolerance may develop readily to drug-induced symptoms having aversive consequences, but little or no tolerance may develop to drug effects having desirable outcomes (Kalant, 1987; Krank, 1989; Stewart, DeWit, & Eikelboom, 1984; Tabakoff & Hoffman, 1988; Wise & Bozarth, 1987). Our theoretical analysis leads to the same view and further suggests that alcohol-induced responses having pleasurable or desirable consequences will be resistant to tolerance unless there is some means of intervening to nullify or remove the desirable consequence.

## Pleasant Expectancies and Alcohol Consumption

Our research on the behavioral effects of alcohol did not examine the influence of alcohol on social drinkers' moods and affective states. Although the consequences of altered emotions under alcohol are more difficult to observe than the consequences of behavior, there is considerable evidence to support the conclusion that affective states induced by alcohol are generally perceived to be pleasant. Drinkers in a North American culture have been found to report that the moods and feelings associated with drinking are expected to yield pleasant outcomes. With respect to feelings, "alcohol is a 'magical' agent that transforms experiences . . . into more positive ones" (Goldman, Brown, & Christiansen, 1987, p. 206).

It also seems likely that the desirability of affective responses to alcohol varies among drinkers. Individuals may differ in their self-perception of feelings and judgments of pleasant emotional states. Diverse social and cultural groups also may convey information leading to different expectations about the pleasant consequences of alcohol-induced feelings. Individual differences in the desirability of the emotional effects of drinking have been observed among subgroups of drinkers in the same culture (Brown, Goldman, & Christiansen, 1985; Worboec et al., 1990). However, the extent to which the expected pleasurable consequences of drinking may be determined by social, cultural, or self-generated information is not known.

Our research demonstrated that the expectation of a desirable consequence for drug-compensatory performance influenced drinkers to alter their behavior to display tolerance under alcohol. An analogous idea has been advanced by the proposal that the expectation of a desirable emotional state under alcohol influences drinkers' behavior with regard to alcohol consumption (Goldman et al., 1987). This "expectancy theory of drinking" suggests that expectancies about the desirable emotional outcomes of drinking determine the self-administration of alcohol. Studies investigating the correlation between the types and intensity of pleasurable emotional consequences and alcohol consumption tend to support the hypothesis. In samples of alcoholics, medical patients and college students, heavier drinkers consistently reported more types of more pleasurable emotional consequences after drinking (Brown et al., 1985). Evidence implying a causative effect of these expectancies has been provided in a 1-year follow-up of drinkers who received treatment for alcoholism. In this sample, those who reported expecting more desirable consequences of drinking were subsequently more likely to drop out of treatment, and to have a poorer treatment outcome (Brown et al., 1985).

The circumstantial nature of these findings is well recognized, and the investigators have noted the need for experimental studies that manipulate the expectation of pleasant outcomes of drinking and show consequent changes in the self-administration of alcohol (Goldman et al., 1987). From our theoretical perspective, such an experiment would be testing the effect of learning the relationship between self-administration of alcohol and a pleasant emotional consequence. In principle, the effects of this expectancy should be as influential as the effect of the Rc-S* expectancy in our studies of behavioral tolerance to alcohol.

## Tolerance: Risks and Benefits

Some time ago, Jellinek (1960) provided a critique of the view that alcohol tolerance increased the risk of excessive drinking. He noted that some investigators considered preexisting innate differences in drinkers' tolerance created the risk, whereas others attributed the risk to tolerance arising through alcohol use. The latter explanation attributes the risk to the development of tolerance to the *pleasant* effects of the drug: "a low to moderate degree of tolerance develops to most of the behavioral and mood-altering effects of alcohol, such that a chronic drinker must take larger and larger amounts in order to obtain the desired effects" (Grilly, 1989, p. 146). Jellinek remained skeptical of the notion that tolerance provided an inducement to increase the use of alcohol, because animal studies had failed to obtain any evidence to support a causal relationship between tolerance and voluntary alcohol consumption. In retrospect, his reservations were well justified. Experiments with animals have not yet successfully shown that tolerance causes an increase in voluntary intake of alcohol, and tolerance to alcohol-induced symptoms that yield pleasant outcomes have not been demonstrated.

The popular assumption that any manifestation of alcohol tolerance creates a risk of excessive drinking remains unproven. Furthermore, the opinion is so widely held that the possibility that some forms of alcohol tolerance may be an asset has not been entertained. Yet this conclusion is clearly suggested by our studies of the development of behavioral tolerance by social drinkers. Their acquisition of tolerance to social doses of alcohol was appropriately adaptive. In general, behavioral tolerance in social drinking situations would seem to have some advantageous consequences. The display of tolerance here would be more beneficial than that of intoxication because tolerant behavior could provide desirable protection from the hazardous consequences of impairment, minimizing not only social disapproval but also accidents in the performance of many tasks such as driving. These generally desirable outcomes of tolerance accruing to social drinkers may explain why it is acquired. From this perspective, a drinker's *failure* to develop behavioral tolerance might be considered abnormal.

## Transition Drinking

The evidence on factors influencing behavioral tolerance in social drinkers provides some speculative clues as to the events that may move a drinker along a path of alcohol abuse that leads to physical dependence. The evidence showed that behavioral tolerance in social drinkers did not necessarily increase with more drinking sessions, or more practice of a task under alcohol. Tolerance was enhanced when the consequence of compensating was more desirable than the consequence of impairment. The opportunity to learn these relationships resulted in tolerance, so that behavior under alcohol was maximally adaptive and ensured the most advantageous outcome. Because social and other environmental consequences can be made contingent upon behavior under alcohol, these expected outcomes should predict whether behavioral tolerance or intoxication is displayed by a social drinker. Thus little or no tolerance should be observed in a situation where symptoms of behavioral intoxication yield a more desirable outcome than compensation.

The same principles may govern emotional responses to alcohol and the attendant perception of the pleasurable consequences of these private internal states. If so, then the development of tolerance here would require the application of some *more desirable* consequence for the *absence* of the pleasurable effects of alcohol. There appears to be no feasible procedure to achieve this. The environmental consequences that induce tolerance to behavioral effects of alcohol cannot readily be made contingent upon unobservable perceptions of pleasure. Thus it seems that desirable mood and emotional consequences of drinking may be quite resistant to tolerance. These speculations suggest that the course of social drinking may result in the acquisition of tolerance to the unwanted behavioral consequences of drinking, and little if any tolerance to the pleasant emotional consequences.

Behavioral tolerance resembles adaptive learning that maximizes the desirable and minimizes the undesirable consequences of a response. The advantageous protection afforded by behavioral tolerance suggests that it may be an extremely common phenomenon, normally acquired by all types of drinkers. The development of behavioral tolerance to alcohol thus seems unlikely to *impel* an increased use of alcohol, but it might offer such an opportunity. If little or no tolerance develops to the pleasurable mood and emotional consequences of drinking, then behavioral tolerance could result in an increased preponderance of desirable over unwanted consequences of drinking. A similar speculation has been advanced by others (Cappell & Le Blanc, 1981; Kalant, 1987). These circumstances presumably would apply to all drinkers. Thus they may account for the wide popularity of alcohol and its use in many cultures over centuries. However, this still would not explain or identify the factors that encourage some social drinkers to make the transition to abusive drinking.

Our notions up to this stage are congruent with conclusions based upon neuropharmacological studies. The evidence suggests that alcohol may resemble opiate and stimulant drugs in activating neural brain mechanisms of reward (Wise, 1988). The incentive systems activated by the drug or drug-associated environmental cues may be comparatively resistant to tolerance (Stewart et al., 1984). This work implies that brain-based affective systems may provide the motivation for maintaining or increasing drug use (Baker, Morse, & Sherman, 1987). However, it also fails to address the question of why the activation of drug-related central incentive systems that motivate alcohol consumption only come to dominate the drinking behavior of some individuals.

The factors responsible for the transition to abusive drinking on the part of some social drinkers are not well understood. Research has tended to search for genetic, or personality, or biological characteristics of a drinker that may increase the risk of alcohol abuse. Particular predisposing characteristics of some drinkers could interact with the effects of alcohol so that the consumption of the drug may have more rewarding consequences. Thus drinkers with such characteristics may increase their alcohol consumption compared with persons without these predisposing attributes. The possibility that environmental factors also may affect drinking behavior is acknowledged, but has received comparatively less research attention. For example, in the investigation of genetic risk factors, Cloninger (1987) identified a Type 1 genetic susceptibility for alcohol abuse that required a "provocative" environment. However, the global indices of environment in the study provided no means of identifying the specific environmental factors that might provoke an increase in alcohol consumption. This knowledge may be crucially important for understanding the factors that encourage the transition from social to abusive drinking.

Studies of drug self-administration in animals show that when different rewards are available for several different activities, animals usually distribute their effort and time so that the maximum number of positive reinforcers is obtained (Domjan & Burkhard, 1986). When positive reinforcements are minimal or unavailable in a situation, the influence of introducing a new rewarding activity, like drug consumption, could come to dominate behavior (Katz & Golberg, 1987; McKim, 1991). Research on social drinkers also shows that their alcohol consumption increases when rewards for alternative behaviors are constrained (Vuchinich & Tucker, 1983; Vuchinich, Tucker, & Rudd, 1987). A recent review of research on this topic concluded that alcohol self-administration emerges as a dominant behavior in an environment that provides sparse rewards, or constrains access to rewards, for alternative behaviors (Vuchinich & Tucker, 1988).

Our analysis would suggest a similar hypothesis. Thus the social drinker who is likely to make the transition to abusive drinking may be the one who expects the emotional effects of alcohol to yield more rewarding outcomes than other activities. Such a preponderance of desirable consequences for drinking behavior may require some predisposing personal characteristics, but any social drinker may be predisposed to increase drinking behavior in an environment where other behaviors offer minimal alternative rewards. Under such circumstances, a drinker may use the opportunity afforded by behavioral tolerance to increase alcohol consumption. An individual who would like to drink more alcohol for its pleasurable consequences on mood and emotion may be enticed to aim to compensate for the impairing behavioral effects of these higher doses. The alluring prospect of drinking more for more pleasurable emotional effects and minimal risk of adverse consequences of behavioral impairment may provide an impetus for escalating consumption. In short, it may be that (1) the *development* of tolerance to the behavioral effects of alcohol simply provides an opportunity to increase the intake of alcohol. (2) the *lack* of tolerance to the pleasurable consequences of drug-induced feelings may provide a motivation for the use of alcohol, and (3) the restricted availability of alternative emotional satisfactions may instigate an increase in consumption

This three-stage proposal concerning the transition to abusive drinking remains to be tested. One implication of our hypotheses is that those who expect more pleasurable effects from drinking should be more likely to use the opportunity afforded by behavioral tolerance to escalate their alcohol consumption. Such a suggestion would be in line with findings on the expected favorable consequences of drinking reported by excessive and social drinkers (Brown, Goldman, Inn, & Anderson, 1980; Goldman et al., 1987; Leigh, 1987). Alcohol abusers do endorse more items in a list of favorable consequences than do social drinkers. This difference in the expectation of desirable consequences of alcohol also appears to begin early in the drinking career, because young problem drinkers are also found to report more favorable consequences than do their social drinking peers. Some research also suggests that these expectations may play a role in instigating excessive drinking. Alcoholics in treatment who reported expecting a greater number of desirable consequences from alcohol have been found to be more prone to relapse after treatment (Brown, 1985). Some investigations of drinkers' rating of the expected intensity of both desirable and unwanted consequences of drinking also point to an overall more favorable expectation on the part of alcohol abusers. Even when social drinkers and abusers expected the same unpleasant consequence, such as hangover, it was rated as less aversive by excessive drinkers (Leigh, 1987).

# Summary

This chapter discussed factors affecting the alcohol tolerance of social drinkers in relationship to the idea that tolerance creates a risk of excessive drinking. Our evidence implies that behavioral tolerance involves perceptual and cognitive processes, with no withdrawal distress that might indicate physical dependence. Social drinkers displayed a remarkable degree of tolerance when the outcome of compensating was more favorable than the consequence of alcohol-induced impairment. Mental or overt training of these response-outcome associations in a situation reliably predicted tolerance. Thus behavioral tolerance to alcohol resembles adaptive learning.

It was suggested that *prior* to the development of physical dependence upon alcohol, tolerance may depend primarily upon learning processes. However, the influence of learning may diminish as continuing exposure to high doses produces physical dependence. At this later stage, tolerance and dependence may be determined primarily by involuntary physiological adaptation to the pharmacological action of the drug.

It appeared that alcohol tolerance should develop whenever a drug-compensatory response provides a more favorable outcome than the consequence of the drug-induced response. Conversely, tolerance may not occur if an alcohol-induced reaction yields a more desirable consequence than the compensatory response. This latter situation appeared likely to apply to the pleasant emotional effects of alcohol, causing them to be very resistant to tolerance. Many observations suggest that the use of alcohol is encouraged by the expectation of pleasant consequences. Because larger doses are needed to overcome tolerance and obtain the initial effect, the impetus for escalating alcohol consumption has often been attributed to the development of tolerance to the pleasant effects of alcohol. Our analysis presented a different perspective on the transition from social to excessive drinking.

Behavioral tolerance is readily acquired by social drinkers and is adaptively advantageous, minimizing hazardous and unwanted consequences of impairment. Thus the *development* of behavioral tolerance per se, seems quite unlikely to impel any increased use of alcohol. The emotionally rewarding effects of drinking may provide a motivation to use alcohol, but this factor also is unlikely to explain the transition from social to abusive drinking because the rewarding consequences of drinking may be comparatively *resistant* to tolerance. Thus the social drinker who is likely to increase the use of alcohol may be the one who expects the emotional effects of alcohol to yield more rewarding outcomes than other activities. Such a preponderance of desirable consequences for drinking behavior may require some predisposing personal characteristics, but any social drinker may be disposed to increase drinking behavior by an environment where other behaviors offer minimal alternative rewards. Under such circumstances, a drinker may use the opportunity afforded by behavioral tolerance to increase alcohol consumption. However, those social drinkers who expect the emotional effects of alcohol to yield more numerous or more intense desirable outcomes could use the opportunity afforded by behavioral tolerance to increase their doses.

Our interpretation of tolerance suggests that the presence or absence of alcohol tolerance may be best predicted by the expectancies that a social drinker has acquired. The evidence on behavioral tolerance has some particularly interesting practical and social ramifications, for it raises the possibility that the responsibility for behavior under alcohol rests more with drinkers and their learning histories than with the action of the drug. These implications are discussed in the next chapter.

# 11

## Social Issues

$\mathbf{A}$s the Introduction stated, understanding how a system normally functions makes identifying and rectifying an abnormality much easier. That outlook is largely reflected in this book. The factors influencing the alcohol tolerance of ordinary social drinkers were first investigated. The information led to suggestions about factors affecting tolerance that might lead to an aberrant increase in the consumption of alcohol. These suggestions, in turn, imply the sorts of interventions that may prevent or ameliorate some of the serious problems that alcohol use and misuse create in society. These strategies are discussed in the present chapter and compared with other approaches that are being tried or advocated.

### Traffic Safety

Most jurisdictions attempt to curb impaired driving by adopting a legal definition of intoxication that makes it an offense to drive a car with a BAC exceeding some moderate level, such as 80 mg/100 ml. By defining lower BACs as legal, this policy implies that they have no hazardous effects on performance. Yet a disproportionate number of alcohol-related car accidents involve young male drivers under mild doses of alcohol, *within* the legal limit (Simpson, 1975). The reason for the overinvolvement of young males in alcohol-related accidents at moderate BACs is not well understood. Current prevention strategies include attempts to protect young adults from alcohol by restricting accessibility (e.g., increasing the cost or raising the legal drinking age). Restricted access policies can only be implemented with the compliance of young social drinkers. Even if the implementation is successful, the strategy is only likely to be effective if moderate doses of alcohol uniformly and uniquely disrupt the performance of young drivers and do not affect those who are a few years older. Few experiments appear to have tested the notion that greater skill on a psychomotor task or more years of drinking experience provide added protection from the impairing effect of mild doses of alcohol. Two studies that have been conducted found no evidence to support these speculations (Beirness & Vogel-Sprott, 1982; Newton, 1978).

A rather different approach to prevention is suggested by the findings on the alcohol tolerance of young adult male social drinkers. These studies demonstrated that resistance to the effect of alcohol was greatly enhanced when the consequence of compensating was more desirable than the consequence of impairment. Recovery during a single dose was hastened, so that the total duration of impairment under the dose was greatly abbreviated. When compensating was associated with a desirable consequence on repeated drinking occasions, the learned expectation of this relationship progressively strengthened tolerance. Impairment often was no longer detectable.

The findings suggest that young drivers may be impaired by moderate doses of alcohol because drug-compensatory driving is not associated with a preferable consequence. Several possible reasons for the absence of such an association could be suggested. Given that society misleadingly implies that moderate BACs are safe because they are legal, young drinkers may have no basis for suspecting that any important degree of impairment will occur, and therefore they may believe no compensation is necessary. It may be that driving is similar to our complex motor skill tasks in that external informative feedback about the adequacy of performance is needed to detect the impairment induced by moderate doses of alcohol. Thus a drinker who wishes to compensate may not do so in the absence of information about the alcohol-induced deficits in skill. Recent evidence suggests that drug-free training of a task under conditions that mimic the impairing effect of alcohol will enhance a drinker's resistance to the effect of moderate BACs the *first* time the task is performed under alcohol (Zinatelli, 1992). Thus alcohol tolerant performance of complex motor tasks may require the expectation of a desirable outcome for compensation *plus* a task-specific compensatory behavioral strategy. Another possibility is that young male drivers perceive compensation to have no particular advantage. Peer group pressure that encourages risk-taking has often been thought to increase the risk of accidents. Membership in such a group also may operate to diminish the desirability of driving with prudent caution under moderate BACs.

These considerations suggest that a reduction in the risk of alcohol-related car accidents at low BACs might be achieved by education. Such a program could alert young drivers to the fact that moderate doses of alcohol can induce impairment, and provide information about the particular deficits in performance that could be anticipated. Given that society adheres to a legal definition of intoxication that allows drinking and driving under some moderate BACs, it seems that society also is obligated to provide training in the driving skills needed to cope with this hazard. Driver training under drug-free conditions that are analogous to alcohol effects (e.g., reduced peripheral vision) could be provided in much the same fashion as current defensive driving programs train drivers to compensate for black ice or other perils that may be encountered. To better insure that the balance of consequences are tipped in favor of compensatory driving, drivers also should be completely informed of the disastrous legal and personal consequences of impaired driving. Stressing the potential advantages of compensating for mild alcohol effects may counteract peer group pressure to court the risk of impairment.

Accident prevention strategies that protect young drivers by restricting their access to alcohol assumes that they are "passive victims" of the drug effect. Our research does not support this assumption. A more promising approach may be an educational program that places the responsibility for behavior under alcohol on the drinker and provides the skill and knowledge to cope. Therefore, young drivers could be able and obligated to control the impairing effect of mild doses of alcohol.

Of course, many car accidents involve drivers with BACs beyond the legal limit. In trying to curb these tragedies, society and the legal system sometimes use mandatory alcoholism treatment and/or stiffer penalties for impaired drivers. It seems that the some combinations of treatment and judicial sanctions could convey a mixed message to drivers concerning the responsibility for the infractions. Treatment is offered to persons who are the victim of an illness, whereas penalties are accorded because of one's own obnoxious behavior. The latter strategy would be more consistent with the educational policy proposed for young drivers and, from our perspective, should be more effective. Comparative studies of the outcome of treatment versus legal prosecution for impaired drivers do find that those who received legal penalties had fewer subsequent accidents and rearrests

(Hagen, Williams, & McConnell, 1979; Preusser, Ulmer, & Adams, 1976; Salzberg & Klingberg, 1983).

## Alcohol Abuse

The terms "alcohol abuse" and "problem drinking" are often used synonymously to refer to the period of alcohol use that intervenes between social drinking and the onset of physical dependence upon alcohol. A very small percentage of alcohol abusers are "alcoholic" in the sense of being physically dependent upon alcohol. When physical dependence occurs, alcoholism is readily diagnosed, and our discussion reserves the term alcoholism for these cases. A diagnosis of alcohol abuse based on judgments of excessive drinking is somewhat unreliable because opinions about what constitutes excessive drinking varies among different cultural and social groups, as well as individuals within the same group. However, a useful indicator of the movement from social to abusive drinking is the onset of social, economic and personal difficulties created by drinkers' behavior under alcohol. The problems typically arise from activities that are readily recognized to violate social or moral standards of conduct, or to create serious physical hazards for the drinker and others. The severity and frequency of these problems may depend upon a drinker's position along the continuum of alcohol abuse. At the social drinking end, behavior under alcohol may generate only occasional slight problems. An example might be unnecessarily rude behavior at a party. As alcohol abuse progresses toward physical dependence, the frequency and severity of problems may increase and involve fatal accidents, assaults, thefts, or murder.

## Drunken Conduct and Responsibility

Research on the determinants of behavioral tolerance in social drinkers might seem far afield from the issues of treatment and prevention of alcohol abuse. Yet the line between social drinkers and abusers is difficult to draw. Like social drinkers, most alcohol abusers are not physically dependent upon alcohol, and abuse is found to vary widely at different times of an individual's life and with different drinking companions. Shifts toward moderation have been correlated with maturation, or life changes that bring alcohol abusers into contact with different people or environments that encourage responsible drinking behavior (Cahalan & Room, 1974; Clark & Cahalan, 1976; Fillmore, 1974).

Our research demonstrated that the display of symptoms of intoxication and tolerance could be controlled by the consequences of a drinker's behavior under alcohol. Alcohol-tolerant behavior was exhibited in drinking situations where it resulted in a more advantageous consequence than intoxicated behavior. In situations where symptoms of intoxication had no penalizing consequence, no tolerance was evident. This evidence showed that behavior under alcohol was not necessarily an inevitable effect of the drug. It was greatly determined by the consequences a drinker had learned to expect for the behavior. The implication for prevention is that society should hold a drinker responsible for his or her behavior and ensure that the consequences are reliable and balanced so that penalties, or at least no advantage, accrues for the display of socially unacceptable behavior.

Many obnoxious, violent and hazardous behaviors are commonly thought to be due to the intoxicating effects of alcohol. An indication of the prevalence of this view is provided by judicial decisions concerning culpability for outrageous behavior under alcohol. In 1985 a Brooklyn man was acquitted of murder, but convicted on the reduced charge of manslaughter, for killing ten people by shots to the head at point-blank range. The defendant was under the influence of drugs at the time, and this extenuating circumstance presumably reduced the charge. " 'It was the drugs,' the jury foreman said" (Rangel, 1985, p. 9). In 1991 a Quebec court judge acquitted a man of sexual assault on the grounds that the defendant was probably too drunk to know what he was doing when he broke into a home and attacked a 65-year-old wheelchair-bound woman.

Our theory suggests that pardoning unacceptable behavior under alcohol fosters the expectation that the behavior is due to the drug. The drinker is thereby excused from responsibility and learns to expect minimal or no adverse consequence for such behavior. A similar view of the attribution of responsibility for drunken behavior has been obtained from historical analyses and legal history (Critchlow, 1983). These considerations imply that drinkers and nondrinkers alike should be accountable for their actions. The social environment presents opportunities to learn the consequences of behavior. Thus the control of unacceptable behavior under alcohol would seem to depend upon the consequences that society provides and leads a drinker to expect.

Such a viewpoint is based upon an extrapolation of evidence on the effect of *moderate* doses of alcohol on *social* drinkers. But it also may apply to higher doses of alcohol, and to drinkers who abuse alcohol. Studies of drinking behavior have demonstrated that alcoholics can exert exquisite control of behavior under extremely high doses of alcohol when the consequences are desirable (Mendelson & Mello, 1966; Nathan, O'Brien, & Lowenstein, 1971). Experiments have also shown that the drinking sprees of dependent alcoholics depend upon their consequences (Nathan, Titler, Lowenstein, Solomon, & Rossi, 1970). These researchers observed that alcoholics who knew when the drinking days would cease gradually reduced their daily consumption prior to the termination in order to minimize their withdrawal symptoms.

Converging evidence implicating the expected consequences of drinking behavior has also been provided by anthropological data on the drinking customs and behavior displayed in different cultures (MacAndrew & Edgerton, 1969). The authors reported that radically different behavioral effects of alcohol were displayed in different societies, but that people within a given culture behaved according to the customs for drunken behavior in their particular social group. The specific behaviors displayed depended upon the cultural sanctions and prohibitions, and these were observed by all members of a given society, even during massive, prolonged intoxication. It seemed that society defined which kinds of behaviors could occur under alcohol, and this conduct became typical. This led to the conclusion that the behavioral effect of *any* amount of alcohol was determined by its consequences. Individuals learn these social consequences, and the behavioral effect of alcohol depends upon what a drinker expects society allows.

## Treatment and Prevention

The transition from social to abusive drinking creates tragic and serious difficulties for many individuals and society at large. Rush (1814) may have been the first to suggest that alcohol abuse may be a disease, but this notion only gained currency during the middle of the 20th century. Jellinek's (1960) classic assessment of the conceptualization of alcoholism as a disease led him to conclude that a disease interpretation was only appropriate to "addicted" drinkers (i.e., those who were physically dependent upon alcohol). He distinguished these drinkers from other "species" in which physical dependence was absent. These latter species are now usually called alcohol abusers or problem drinkers. Although Jellinek's notion of a disease process in alcoholism was narrowly restricted to physical dependence, the disease concept is currently widely generalized to drinkers who have problems related to alcohol use prior to physical dependence. These are the persons who are termed alcohol abusers. They greatly outnumber the drinkers who are physically dependent, and are the ones to which our research findings might be most appropriately extrapolated.

Most strategies for the prevention and treatment of alcoholism in North America are influenced by the disease concept. The view of alcohol abuse as a disease acquired by the ingestion of alcohol dictates the sort of treatment needed. Because alcohol apparently instigates the disease, the individual is not held responsible for falling ill, but abstinence is mandatory to halt the disease and protect the patient. The progressive nature of a disease has also led to the view that subtle problems arising from drinking behavior may grow unless checked. Thus early-stage treatments should be offered to drinkers who have *any* problems. There is also an obligation to help individuals at risk for contracting the disease, before any symptoms are manifest. Such a view has encouraged the search for genetic or other biological "markers" of a predisposition to abuse alcohol among family members of alcoholics. A massive study of the genetics of alcoholism, involving hundreds of alcoholics and their family members is now underway (Holden, 1991). Several prevention policies consistent with reducing the spread of a disease are also in place. Some examples are pricing policies, the control of the distribution and sale of alcoholic beverages, and server intervention programs where bartenders are liable for the intoxicated behavior of their patrons. The implication here is that drinkers are not themselves able to resist alcohol abuse or the behavioral effect of the drug. The drinker must depend upon society for protection from alcohol and accept treatment when the disease strikes.

Skepticism of the concept of alcoholism as a disease has increased in recent years (Fingarette, 1988; Faulkner, Sandage, & Maguire, 1988; Peele, 1989). Some criticism stems from objections to its "passive victim" implication. Peele (1989) has argued that by identifying the drug as the problem, the disease concept reinforces and excuses alcoholism. It convinces people that they cannot control their own behavior and pardons their outrageous conduct. Peele considers that alcoholism refers to

> people who get drunk more than other people and who often suffer problems due to their drinking . . . overdrinking, compulsive

drinking, drinking beyond a point where the person knows he or
she will regret it. . . . It happens to quite a high percentage of all
drinkers during their lives. (1989, p. 60)

According to Peele, alcoholism and alcohol abuse are synonymous,
and there is no disease.

> Alcoholics are no different from other human beings in exercising
> choices, seeking the feelings that they believe alcohol provides, and
> in evaluating the mood changes they experience in terms of their
> alternatives . . . alcoholics continue to respond to their environ-
> ments and to express personal values even while they are drinking.
> (1989, p. 60)

Enthusiasm for the disease concept of alcoholism also has been
tempered by the implications of searching for, and helping young
individuals at risk for alcohol abuse by virtue of their genetic makeup
or heritable traits. Evidence that *something* transmitted genetically
influences later development of alcoholism has been furnished by
adoption studies (Goodwin, Schulsinger, Hermansen, Guze, & Winokur, 1973; Schuckit, Goodwin, & Winokur, 1972a, 1972b). Sons of
alcoholics are found to have a higher incidence of alcoholism than
sons of nonalcoholic parents. Male children with a family history of
alcoholism are estimated to have a 24% incidence of alcoholism. This
means that 76% of these individuals do *not* develop alcoholism. Thus
preventative interventions with sons of alcoholics may be unnecessary in 76% of the cases, and would miss alcoholic sons of nonalcoholic parents (Fingarette, 1988).

Although the incidence of alcoholism among groups can be
estimated, *individuals* at risk cannot yet be adequately identified.
Cloninger, Sigvardsson, and Bohman (1988) have provided evidence
for an association between particular personality traits of children and
their development of alcoholism in adulthood. However, these
investigators note that the childhood criteria that successfully predict
the incidence of alcoholism for a group would give the wrong
prediction in 74% of cases that an individual is predicted to be
alcoholic. The possibility that research may succeed in locating
molecular or other genetic markers for those at risk of alcoholism also
raises ethical questions (Wilson & Crowe, in press). The young
people so identified would be asymptomatic, but their identification
would necessarily obligate the imposition of some treatment to
prevent them from contracting alcohol abuse. However, such interventions applied to individuals with no behavioral signs of alcohol

abuse could violate ethical principles of autonomy and privacy, and lead to discrimination on the basis of genetic makeup.

Other reservations have been prompted by disappointing results of alcoholism treatment. Research and reviews of treatment outcomes by adherents of a disease model and its medical treatment have led to the conclusion that "there is compelling evidence that the results of our treatment were no better than the natural history of the disease" (Vaillant, 1983, pp. 283–284). On the question of what increased the likelihood of remission, Vaillant concluded, "The most important single prognostic variable among alcoholics who received treatment was having something to lose if they continued to abuse alcohol" (1983, p. 188). It seems that drinkers recovered from alcohol abuse when changes in their life circumstances made it worthwhile to reduce their consumption, and when these rewards exceeded and counteracted those obtained with alcohol.

To the extent that such a surmise is correct, it points to the *consequences* of drinking as an important determinant of treatment outcome. Such a view is consistent with findings reviewed in previous chapters. Our research demonstrated that the consequences of behavior under alcohol could predict tolerance. A drinker displayed tolerance when it yielded a more desirable outcome than the symptoms of alcohol intoxication. The tolerance-inducing effect of the behavioral consequences suggested their role in encouraging an increased use of alcohol may be to increase the preponderance of pleasurable consequences of alcohol. Given that tolerance is readily acquired to unwanted behavioral effects but not to pleasant emotional effects of alcohol, the preponderance of desirable consequences could increase. Thus drinkers at risk of escalating their consumption might be those who find other activities yield consequences that are not sufficiently desirable to compete with those obtained from alcohol. This interpretation implies that programs to treat and prevent alcohol abuse should consider the consequences of a drinker's reactions to alcohol.

The expectation that drinking yields the most desirable consequences is likely to be well established by the time alcohol abuse becomes evident and treatment is attempted. After such an expectancy has been learned, it may be very difficult to alter. Personal perceptions of feelings cannot be repressed by external forces, and a drinker's resources for change may be limited by the absence of alternative activities to substitute for the pleasurable consequences of alcohol use. Disease-oriented treatment programs typically insist on abstinence. Although the prohibition of alcohol would guarantee the absence of alcohol abuse, high relapse rates show that abstinence is difficult to enforce. From our perspective, compelling abstinence may repress the *expression* of drug-taking but is unlikely to change the expected satisfactions of drinking. To the extent that these expectations initiate the consumption of alcohol, they may instigate a relapse when the opportunity to drink becomes available. This viewpoint suggests that treatment to counteract abusive drinking should include the training of alternative responses to situations where excessive drinking has occurred. Here the acquisition of new behaviors to access other rewards may provide an individual with new coping behavior and the opportunity to perceive that the total joy and satisfactions gained from alternative activities can equal or exceed those derived from drinking.

Some treatment strategies that include an assessment of the expectancies and behavior associated with drinking have been proposed. The relapse prevention program developed by G. Alan Marlatt and colleagues at the University of Washington is a notable example (Marlatt & Gordon, 1985). This approach trains new coping skills that substitute for excessive drinking. The identification of the skills needed by a problem drinker is based upon an assessment of the conditions and expectancies associated with the occurrence and maintenance of drinking. The evidence suggests that this assessment provides a good indication of appropriate and effective training strategies and predicts the treatment outcome (Donovan & Marlatt, 1980). The efficacy of this treatment approach in reducing the preference for drinking may derive in part from the learning of social skills that increase a drinker's ability to attain rewards that were previously unavailable (Vuchinich & Tucker, 1988).

A similar perspective is evident in some prevention strategies. The training of new coping skills and adaptive social behavior has been advocated as a means of preventing substance abuse by youths (Brown & Mills, 1987). Studies have shown that social drinkers cannot accurately identify their own BACs (Beirness, 1987). A great many drinkers *underestimate* their blood alcohol levels. Thus responsible drinkers may not have the information needed to comply with a law that defines intoxication by a particular BAC. However, research on training BAC estimation has shown that accurate discrimination of moderate BACs can be learned by light and heavy social drinkers (Bois & Vogel-Sprott, 1974, 1975; Ogurzsoff & Vogel Sprott, 1976). Training in self-regulation of alcohol consumption has been proposed as a means of increasing responsible drinking behavior and reducing impaired driving (Worden et al., 1989). A recent study has examined the efficacy of a prevention program that provided training in BAC estimation, identification of alcohol-related expectancies, responsible decision-making and coping skills for maintaining self-imposed limits to drinking (Kivlahan, Marlatt, Fromme, Coppel, & Williams 1990). College students whose high alcohol consumption placed them at risk of immediate and long-term alcohol-related problems were randomly assigned to the prevention program, or didactic alcohol information, or a control condition. Follow-up measures of drinking, obtained at 4, 8, and 12 months, showed a decline in alcohol consumption that consistently favored the group receiving the prevention program.

The underlying assumptions inherent in such treatment and prevention programs are consistent with the implications of our research. Together they point to the conclusion that halting and preventing alcohol abuse is the responsibility of both the person and society. A drinker is ultimately accountable for his or her drinking behavior. But it is influenced by the consequences that drinkers have learned to expect from alcohol, and society has a major influence on, and responsibility for, training these expectancies.

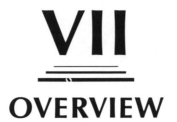

# OVERVIEW

# 12

## Alcohol, Science, and Society

This book has described experiments on alcohol tolerance that are similar to other investigations in that tolerance was inferred from a diminished response to a dose, and tolerance was assumed to reflect the occurrence of a drug-compensatory response that opposed the drug effect. However, the results of our investigations are at odds with many widely accepted theories and conclusions about the determinants of alcohol tolerance.

There are several reasons for the uniqueness of our findings. Most of the information and conclusions pertaining to alcohol tolerance have been derived from the administration of fairly large doses to animals or to alcoholics. In contrast, our findings are based upon the administration of moderate doses of alcohol to young adults at the beginning of their social drinking careers. The systematic collection of this type of evidence has not previously been presented. Further, investigations of alcohol tolerance have typically examined the effect of drug exposures, or of environmental events reliably associated with the administration of alcohol. The latter research has identified a learning component in tolerance, a "stimulus expectancy for drug" that allows a subject to anticipate the occurrence of a drug. Our studies were designed to hold these particular variables constant so as to test the impact on tolerance of events *after* a dose of alcohol is received.

We proposed that events related to behavior under alcohol could introduce information leading to an additional influential learned expectancy concerning the association between a drinker's behavior and its consequence. The experiments consistently suggested that the association of a drug-compensatory response with a desirable consequence greatly enhanced tolerance and predicted the strength of a drug-opposite compensatory response when drinkers subsequently expected alcohol but received a placebo. Moreover, tolerance was only enhanced in situations where individuals had an opportunity to learn to expect an advantageous consequence for compensating. Repetitions of this association increased tolerance. In addition, tolerance could be enhanced by repeated *mental* rehearsal of compensatory performance and a favorable outcome, or by repetitions of this association during overt performance. Thus it appeared that information about the consequences of behavior under alcohol could be perceived by a drinker without firsthand experience of the response-outcome events.

In contrast to surveys that examine correlations between individuals' expectancies and their alcohol-related behavior, our research tested causal effects. Thus our investigations of the influence of expectancies on alcohol tolerance took the form of experiments that controlled other possible tolerance-inducing factors, such as alcohol exposures, expectation of alcohol, and task practice. Psychomotor skill tasks were chosen for examination for two reasons: Social drinkers often perform these sorts of tasks under alcohol, and individual differences in prior familiarity with a task could be controlled by using tasks that drinkers had not performed prior to an experiment. Demonstrations that the expected consequences of behavior under alcohol reliably affected tolerance led to a host of interesting questions about the generality of the results, the predictive scope of the theory, and possible practical applications to the treatment and prevention of alcohol abuse.

The discussion of the implications of the findings adopted Jellinek's (1960) view that the disease concept of alcoholism may only pertain to drinkers who are addicted, that is, physically dependent upon alcohol. The term *alcohol abuse* was used to refer to problem drinkers prior to the onset of physical dependence. In contrast to a disease concept that emphasizes the risk induced by alcohol, research in this book called attention to the important additional insights that can be gained by a systematic investigation of relationships between alcohol, behavior and its consequence that drinkers learn to expect.

A behavioral approach to questions about alcohol effects and the puzzle of alcohol abuse is no substitute for the knowledge and understanding of the physiological, neurochemical, and pharmacological effects of alcohol. The contribution of behavioral science is to highlight a different facet of alcohol-related problems: to show that the responsibility for solutions rests with individuals and society as well as the biomedical sciences.

What appears to be needed are studies that systematically examine alcohol abuse in relationship to the setting and to the emotional and behavioral consequences of alcohol use. A continuation of this approach with social drinking promises to contribute to our understanding of factors responsible for the maintenance of moderate drinking and the transition to abusive drinking. It is ironic to note that the need for such research was perceived so long ago by Jellinek himself, when he warned against an overinclusive conceptualization of alcoholism as a disease.

> If the formulation rigidly claims that alcohol addiction or any other species of alcoholism is purely a medical problem, any preventive attempt may be seriously impaired. The usefulness of the idea . . . depends, to a large extent, upon the recognition of social and economic factors in the etiology of all species of alcoholism. By the recognition of these factors I do not mean mere assent that such factors exist but exploration and understanding of them. . . . There remains the fact that a learning theory of drinking in the well-defined terms of psychological discipline is essential to all species of alcoholism, including addiction. (1960, pp. 158, 77)

# *Appendices*

## APPENDIX A
### Recommended Menu for Alcohol Sessions

Eat a light meal followed by *3.5 hours of fasting* before you come to your appointment. For example, if your appointment is at 4:00 p.m., have a light snack at about 12:00 p.m. and then eat nothing for 3.5 hours. Below is a list of suggested foods and a list of foods to avoid. In general, avoid all dairy products and all greasy, fried foods (e.g., anything with butter). Thank you for your cooperation.

*Suggested foods:*
- breads, buns, muffins
- fruits, vegetables
- seafood (nothing packed in oil)
- meat or poultry (broiled, baked, or barbecued)
- hard or soft boiled eggs
- toast with jam (no butter)
- salad (no dressing)
- sandwiches (luncheon meats, with mustard only)
- soup (not creamed)
- pickles

*Foods to avoid:*
- all dairy products (e.g., cheese, butter, yogurt, ice cream, margarine, or milk)
- mayonnaise
- fried eggs
- fried hamburgers
- french fries, chips
- bacon
- donuts
- peanut butter

*Beverages:*
- coffee, tea (keep to a minimum)
- juice, soda

- Please do not skip this light meal 4 hours before a session.

- Please do not take any prescription or nonprescription drugs. Notify the experimenter if you have taken any prescripion or nonprescription drugs (such as aspirin or cold medication for a headache or cold).

NO ALCOHOL OR OTHER RECREATIONAL DRUGS 24 HOURS BEFORE A DRINKING SESSION.

## APPENDIX B
### Personal Drinking History Questionnaire

Below are some questions that are primarily concerned with your personal history of drinking. Most ask you to answer according to what is most typical or usual for you. Please try to answer each question as honestly as possible.

Age: _____   Weight: _____ lb or _____ kg
Height: _____ in or _____ cm

1. How long have you been drinking alcohol on a regular basis?
    a. _____ months
    b. _____ years

2. How often, on average, do you drink alcohol socially, that is, with others? (Choose only one.)
    a. Only on special occasions _____ How many times per year? _____
    b. Monthly, how often? _____
    c. Weekly, how often? _____
    d. Daily, how often? _____

3. What alcoholic beverage do you prefer? _____

4. What alcoholic beverage do you usually drink? _____

5. In terms of the beverage indicated in question 4, what is the *average* quantity you drink in a single drinking occasion? (Choose only one.)
    a. Wine (estimate ounces)
        1  2  3  4  5  6  7  8  9  10 or _____
    b. Beer (bottles)
        1  2  3  4  5  6  7  8  9  10 or _____
    c. Beer (draft glasses)
        1  2  3  4  5  6  7  8  9  10 or _____
    d. Liquor (assume 1.5 oz per drink and estimate number of drinks)
        1  2  3  4  5  6  7  8  9  10 or _____
6. How long does your typical drinking session last? (Choose one only.)
    a. _____ minutes
    b. _____ hours
    c. _____ days

*Scoring Instructions*

*Frequency* of drinking was calculated as the number of times per week the individual reported consuming alcohol.

*Dose* was defined as volume of absolute alcohol (ml) per kg body weight consumed on a typical drinking occasion. Total ml of absolute alcohol was determined by multiplying the number of drinks (in ml) reported to be consumed on a typical drinking occasion by the concentration of alcohol in the particular beverage. Beer was taken as 5% alcohol by volume, liquor 40%, and wine 15%. A bottle of beer contains 341 ml; therefore, 341 × 5% = 17.045 ml of absolute alcohol. The total ml of alcohol was then divided by body weight in kg to produce a dose score for each subject.

*Duration of a drinking occasion* was measured in hours.

*Rate of consumption* was calculated by dividing dose by the length of a typical drinking occasion in hours. This dose-per-hour measure is intended to give a better representation of the concentration of alcohol in the body in a given period of time than would dose alone.

Mean Drinking Habit Scores from 100 Male Subjects in Eperiments by Beirness (1983), Mann (1980), and Sdao-Jarvie (1988)

| Age (yr) | Dose (ml/kg) | Frequency (per wk) | Duration (hr) | Drink rate (dose/duration) |
|----------|--------------|--------------------|---------------|----------------------------|
| 20.6     | 1.20*        | 2.44               | 3.01          | 0.45                       |

Mean Drinking Habit Scores from a Survey of 533 Male University of Waterloo Students (Chipperfield & Vogel-Sprott, 1984)

| Age (yr) | Dose (ml/kg) | Frequency (per wk) | Duration (hr) | Drink rate (dose/duration) |
|----------|--------------|--------------------|---------------|----------------------------|
| 21       | 1.14**       | 1.44               | 3.82          | 0.30                       |

Dose per occasion can be estimated in beer by multiplying a drinker's dose by kg body weight and dividing by 17.045 (i.e., the alcohol in a 341-ml bottle of 5% beer).
*Assuming a body weight of 70 kg, the dose equals 4.9 bottles of beer.
**Assuming a body weight of 70 kg, the dose equals 4.7 bottles of beer.
The national survey of a representative sample of Canadians by Nutrition Canada (1973) included 2,541 male drinkers. The data indicated that 95% of men 21–25 years of age reported doses of 1.20 ml/kg or less (i.e., equivalent to 4.9 bottles of beer per occasion).

## APPENDIX C
## Psychomotor Tasks

*The Tracometer Task*

This subject-paced tracking task was developed and built by the National Research Council of Canada (Buck, Leonardo, & Hyde, 1981). To perform the task, a subject sits before a vertical target display panel and grasps a steering wheel with both hands. The steering wheel controls a pointer that moves across the target display panel. The Plexiglas pointer has a hairline cross that must be centered over a target on the panel. Although the ratio of wheel-to-pointer movement is 1:1, the task is fairly difficult because the two components move in opposite directions. The target display panel contains five 2.4-mm circles, each separated by a distance of 41 mm. Whenever a circle is illuminated, it serves as a target. When a subject's pointer is correctly aligned over a target for an uninterrupted period of 200 milliseconds, a new target is illuminated in one of the other four positions. The machine could be programmed to present, or withhold, a pleasant auditory signal whenever a target is hit.

A single test presents 100 targets. The order of target presentations on each test is varied according to one of ten predetermined sequences. Each sequence begins with the center target position, and continues so that each of 20 possible movements between pairs of targets occurs five times.

A control unit, outside the subject's range of vision, counts each target and records the number of movement errors, the speed of several component movements involved in the performance of the task, and a composite measure of overall speed (i.e., total time to complete a test). A moderate dose of alcohol has been found to depress all measures of speed of tracometer performance and to leave errors unaffected (Beirness & Vogel-Sprott, 1982). Therefore, the best evaluation of alcohol effects on task performance is provided by the composite speed score, total time to complete a test.

*Pursuit Rotor Task*

To perform this task, a subject is seated at a small table in front of a box, 40 cm square and 13 cm high. A glass plate on the top of the box presents a frosted track, 15.5 cm square and 1.5 mm wide, on a black background. A beam of light, visible beneath the frosted square, rotates clockwise at 30 rpm. The subject is required to track the light with a photosensitive stylus, held in the preferred hand. A test on the task takes about 3 minutes and consists of two 50-second practice periods, separated by a 30-second rest. A millisecond timer automatically records the time the stylus is in contact with the light beam. This time-on-target (TOT) score measures performance of the task.

The pursuit rotor is commercially available (Lafayette Instrument Company—Model 30014). It rotates the light target on a mechanical turntable. A replica built at the University of Waterloo eliminated the turntable by substituting light-emitting diodes (LEDs) programmed to give the illusion of a moving light target beneath the track. Both types of pursuit rotor equipment were modified by the installation of a signaling device that could be activated to provide a soft buzz (1,000 Hz, 72 dB maximum) whenever the subject's stylus was in contact with the light target.

# APPENDIX D
## Instruments to Measure BAC from Breath Samples


Several instruments to estimate BAC from breath samples are commercially available. The ones used in our laboratory are:

- the Breathalyser (Stephenson Instrument Co.)
- an Intoxilizer (Omicron Systems Inc.)
- a BAC Verifier (Verax Ltd.)

The Breathalyser depends upon a wet chemical method of analysis. The Intoxilizer and the BAC Verifier each use an infrared ray refraction process and provide an instantaneous digital readout of the BAC measure. All three types of instruments have comparable accuracy, but the determination of BAC by the Breathalyser is slower and less convenient.

## APPENDIX E
## Example Tape Transcript of Mental Rehearsal Instructions

*To Guide a 50-Second Mental Rehearsal Trial on the Pursuit Rotor*

As you imagine yourself performing the task, I want you to relax and try to make your images as vivid as possible. Try to shut out all external distractions and concentrate on your mental images.

First, I want you to imagine that you are sitting in front of the pursuit rotor . . . try to mentally picture the pursuit rotor . . . try to see the stylus and target area of the pursuit rotor. Now imagine yourself preparing to perform the task. Imagine yourself picking up the stylus . . . try to feel the stylus in your hand. Next, imagine yourself putting the stylus in the starting position in the center pattern, ready to begin the trial . . . try to feel your arm move as you do this. Next, visualize the light moving around the target area in a clockwise direction. Imagine yourself moving the stylus in order to track the light. For the next 50 seconds, imagine yourself trying to track the light over an entire trial.

*(The next three comments occur at approximately 15-second intervals.)* Try to feel your arm move as you continue to track the light with the stylus . . . Try to picture yourself accurately tracking the light with the stylus. . . . Imagine yourself tracking the light with the stylus.

*(Comment at 50 seconds.)* Finally, mentally evaluate your performance during the trial. . . . If your imaginary performance equaled or bettered your criterion performance, try to identify what you did to achieve it. . . . If your imaginary performance did not equal or better your criterion performance, try to identify the mistakes you made that prevented you from achieving your criterion.

# References

American Psychiatric Association. (1987). *Diagnostic and statistical manual of mental disorders* (3rd ed., rev.). Washington, DC: Author.

Annear, W. C., & Vogel-Sprott, M. (1985). Mental rehearsal and classical conditioning contribute to ethanol tolerance in humans. *Psychopharmacology, 87*, 90–93.

Baker, T. B., Morse, E., & Sherman, J. E. (1987). The motivation to use drugs: A psychobiological analysis of urges. In P. C. Rivers (Ed.), *Nebraska symposium on motivation: Vol. 34. Alcohol and addictive behavior* (pp. 257–323). Lincoln: University of Nebraska Press.

Barrett, J. E., Glowa, J. R., & Nader, M. A. (1989). Behavioral and pharmacological history as determinants of tolerance and sensitization-like phenomena in drug action. In A. J. Goudie & M. W. Emmett-Oglesby (Eds.), *Psychoactive drugs: tolerance and sensitization* (pp. 181–219). Clifton, NJ: Humana.

Beirness, D. J. (1983). *Reinforcement contingencies control the development of behavioural tolerance in social drinkers.* Unpublished PhD thesis, University of Waterloo, Waterloo, Ontario.

Beirness, D. J. (1987). Self-estimates of blood alcohol concentration in drinking–driving context. *Drug and Alcohol Dependence, 19*, 79–90.

Beirness, D. J., & Vogel-Sprott, M. (1982). Does prior skill reduce alcohol-induced impairment? *Journal of Studies on Alcohol, 43*, 1149–1156.

Beirness, D. J., & Vogel-Sprott, M. (1984a). Alcohol tolerance in social drinkers: Operant and classical conditioning effects. *Psychopharmacology, 84*, 393–397.

Beirness, D. J., & Vogel-Sprott, M. (1984b). The development of alcohol tolerance: Acute recovery as a predictor. *Psychopharmacology, 84*, 398–401.

Blodgett, H. C. (1929). The effect of the introduction of reward upon the maze performance of rats. *University of California Publications in Psychology, 5,* 113–134.

Boakes, R. A. (1989). How one might find evidence for conditioning in adult humans. In T. Archer & L. Nilsson (Eds.), *Aversion, avoidance, and anxiety: Perspectives on aversively motivated behavior* (pp. 381–402). Hillsdale, NJ: Erlbaum.

Bois, C., & Vogel-Sprott, M. (1974). Discrimination of low blood alcohol levels and self-titration skills in social drinkers. *Quarterly Journal of Studies on Alcohol, 35,* 86–97.

Bolles, R. C. (1972). Reinforcement, expectancy and learning. *Psychological Review, 79,* 394–409.

Bolles, R. C. (1975). *Theory of motivation* (2nd ed.). New York: Harper & Row.

Bolles, R. C. (1979). *Learning theory* (2nd ed.). New York: Holt, Rinehart and Winston.

Branch, M. N. (1983). Behavioral tolerance to the stimulating effects of pentobarbital: A within-subject determination. *Pharmacology, Biochemistry and Behavior, 18,* 25–30.

Branch, M. N. (1984). Rate dependency, behavioral mechanisms, and behavioral pharmacology. *Journal of the Experimental Analysis of Behavior, 42,* 511–522.

Brewer, W. F. (1974). There is no convincing evidence for operant and classical conditioning in human beings. In W. B. Weimer & D. J. Palermo (Eds.), *Cognition and the symbolic processes* (pp. 1–42). Hillsdale, NJ: Erlbaum.

Britton, K. T., Ehlers, C. L., & Koob, G. F. (1988). Is ethanol antagonist Ro15-4513 selective for ethanol? *Science, 239,* 648–649.

Brocco, M. J., Rastogi, S. K., & McMillan, D. E. (1983). Effects of chronic phencyclidine (PCP) on the schedule controlled behaviour of rats. *Journal of Pharmacology and Experimental Therapeutics, 226,* 449–454.

Brown, B., & Mills, A. R. (Eds.). (1987). *Youth at high risk for substance abuse.* Rockville, MD: National Institute on Drug Abuse.

Brown, S. A. (1985). Reinforcement expectancies and alcohol treatment outcome after a one year followup. *Journal of Studies on Alcohol, 46,* 304–308.

Brown, S. A., Goldman, M. S., & Christiansen, B. A. (1985). Do alcohol expectancies mediate drinking patterns of adults? *Journal of Consulting and Clinical Psychology, 53,* 512–519.

Brown, S., Goldman, M., Inn, A., & Anderson, L. (1980). Expectations of reinforcement from alcohol: Their domain and relation to drinking patterns. *Journal of Consulting and Clinical Psychology, 48,* 419–426.

Buck, L. R., Leonardo, R., & Hyde, F. (1981). Measuring performance with the NRC "stressalyzer." *Applied Ergonomics, 12,* 231–236.

Cahalan, D., & Room, R. (1974). *Problem drinking among American men.* New Brunswick, NJ: Rutgers Center of Alcohol Studies.

Campo, R. A. (1973). Development of tolerance in pigeons to the behavioral effects of a new benzopyran derivative. *Journal of Pharmacology and Experimental Therapeutics, 184,* 521–527.

Cappell, H., & LeBlanc, A. (1979). Tolerance to, and physical dependence on, ethanol: Why do we study them? *Drug and Alcohol Dependence, 4,* 15–31.

Cappell, H., Roach, C., & Poulos, C. X. (1981). Pavlovian cross-tolerance between pentobarbital and ethanol. *Psychopharmacology, 74,* 54–57.

Carder, B., & Olson, J. (1973). Learned behavioral tolerance to marihuana in rats. *Pharmacology, Biochemistry and Behavior, 1,* 73–76.

Carpenter, J. A. (1962). Effects of alcohol on some psychological processes. *Quarterly Journal of Studies on Alcohol, 23,* 274–314.

Chen, C. S. (1968). A study of the alcohol tolerance effect and an introduction of a new behavioral technique. *Psychopharmacologia, 12,* 433–440.

Chen, C. S., (1972). A further note on studies of acquired behavioral tolerance to alcohol. *Psychopharmacologia, 27,* 265–274.

Chen, C. S. (1979). Acquisition of behavioral tolerance to ethanol as a function of reinforced practice in rats. *Psychopharmacology, 63,* 285–288.

Chin, J. H., & Goldstein, D. (1981). Membrane-disordering action of ethanol. *Molecular Pharmacology, 19,* 425–431.

Chipperfield, B., & Vogel-Sprott, M. (1984). Student's drinking habits and family history of problem drinking (Abstract No. 96). *Canadian Psychology, 25* (2a).

Clark, W., & Cahalan, D. (1976. Changes in problem drinking over a four year span. *Addictive Behaviors, 1,* 251–259.

Cloninger, C. R. (1987). Neurogenetic adaptive mechanisms in alcoholism. *Science, 236,* 410–416.

Cloninger, C. R., Sigvardsson, S., & Bohman, M. (1988). Childhood personality predicts alcohol abuse in young adults. *Alcoholism: Clinical and Experimental Research, 12,* 494–505.

Coldwell, B. B., & Smith, H. W. (1959). Alcohol levels in body fluids after ingestion of distilled spirits. *Canadian Journal of Biochemistry, 37,* 43–52.

Collier, H. O. J. (1965). A general theory of the genesis of drug dependence by induction of receptors. *Nature, 205,* 181–182.

Collins, R. L., & Searles, J. S. (1988). Alcohol and the balanced placebo design: Were experimenter demands in expectancy really tested? Comment on Knight, Barbaree, and Boland (1986). *Journal of Abnormal Psychology, 97,* 503–507.

Colwill, R. M., & Rescorla, R. A. (1986). Associative structures in instrumental learning. In G. H. Bower (Ed.), *The psychology of learning and motivation* (Vol. 20, pp. 55–104). New York: Academic Press.

Corbin, C. B. (1972) Mental practice. In W. P. Morgan (Ed.), *Ergogenic aids and muscular performance* (pp. 93–118). New York: Academic Press.

Corfield-Sumner, P. K., & Stolerman, J. P. (1978). Behavioral tolerance. In D. Blackman & D. Sanger (Eds.), *Contemporary research in behaviorial pharmacology* (pp. 391–448). New York: Plenum.

Critchlow, B. (1983). Blaming the booze: The attribution of responsibility for drunken behavior. *Personality and Social Psychology Bulletin, 9,* 451–473.

Crowell, C. R., Hinson, R. E., & Siegel, S. (1981). The role of conditioned drug responses to the hypothermic effects of ethanol. *Psychopharmacology, 73,* 51–54.

Dafters, R., & Anderson, G. (1982). Conditioned tolerance to the tachycardia effect of ethanol in humans. *Psychopharmacology, 78,* 365–367.

de Souza Moreira, L. F., Caprigliore, M. J., & Masur, J. (1981). Development and reacquisition of tolerance to ethanol administered pre- and posttrials to rats. *Psychopharmacology, 73,* 165–167.

Dews, P. B. (1955). Studies on behavior: Differential sensitivity to pentobarbital of pecking performance in pigeons depending on the schedule of reward. *Journal of Pharmacology and Experimental Therapeutics, 113,* 393–401.

Dews, P. B. (1962). Psychopharmacology. In A. J. Bachrach (Ed.), *Foundations of clinical psychology* (pp. 423–441). New York: Basic Books.

DiPadova, D., Worner, T. M., Julkunen, R., & Lieber, C. (1987). Effects of fasting and chronic alcohol consumption on the first-pass metabolism of ethanol. *Gastroenterology, 92,* 1169–1173.

Domjan, M., & Burkhard, B. (1986). *The principles of learning and behavior* (2nd ed.). Monterey, CA: Brooks/Cole.

Donovan, D., & Marlatt, G. A. (1980). Assessment of expectancies and behaviors associated with alcohol consumption. *Journal of Studies on Alcohol, 41,* 1153–1185.

Druckman, D., & Swetz, J. (Eds.) (1988). *Enhancing human performance: Issues, theories and techniques.* Washington, DC: National Academic Press.

Duncan, D., & Vogel-Sprott, M. (1978). Drinking habits of impaired drivers. *Blutalkohol, 15,* 252–260.

Egger, M. D., & Miller, N. E. (1962). Secondary reinforcement in rats as a function of information value and reliability of the stimulus. *Journal of Experimental Psychology, 64,* 97–104.

Egstrom, G. (1964). Effects of an emphasis on conceptualizing techniques during early learning of a gross motor skill. *Research Quarterly, 35,* 472–481.

Eikelboom, R., & Stewart, J. (1982). Conditioning of drug-induced physiological responses. *Psychological Review, 89,* 509–528.

Elsmore, T. F. (1976). The role of reinforcement loss in tolerance to chronic THC effects on the operant behavior of rhesus monkeys. *Pharmacology, Biochemistry and Behavior, 5,* 123–128.

Engel, R., Paskaruk, S., & Green, N. (1978). *Driver education evaluation tests: Summary report.* Toronto: Ministry of Transport.

Faulkner, W., Sandage, D., & Maguire, B. (1988) The disease concept of alcoholism: The persistence of an outmoded scientific paradigm. *Deviant Behavior, 9,* 317–332.

Feltz, D., & Landers, D. (1983). The effects of mental practice on motor skill learning and performance: A meta-analysis. *Journal of Sport Psychology, 5,* 25–57.

Ferraro, D. P., & Grilly, D. M. (1973). Lack of tolerance to delta-9-THC in chimpanzees. *Science, 179,* 490.

Fillmore, K. M. (1974). Drinking and problem drinking in early adulthood and middle age. *Quarterly Journal of Studies on Alcohol, 35,* 819–840.

Fillmore, M. (1990). *Predicting a placebo response: The role of expectancies concerning drug effects.* Unpublished MASc thesis, University of Waterloo, Waterloo, Ontario.

Fillmore M., & Vogel-Sprott, M. (1992). Expected effect of caffeine on motor performance predicts the type of response to placebo. *Psychopharmacology, 106*(2), 209–214.

Fingarette, H. (1988). *Heavy drinking: The myth of drinking as a disease.* Berkeley: University of California Press.

Forney, R. B., & Harger, R. N. (1971). The alcohols. In J. R. DiPalma (Ed.), *Drill's pharmacology in medicine* (4th ed., pp. 275–302). New York: McGraw-Hill.

Frankel, D., Khanna, J. M., Kalant, H., & LeBlanc, A. (1978). Effect of *p*-chlorophenylalanine on the loss and maintenance of tolerance to ethanol. *Psychopharmacology, 56*, 139–144.

Frezza, M., di Padova, C., Pozzato, G., Terpin, M., Barona, E., & Lieber, C. S. (1990). High blood alcohol levels in women: The role of decreased gastric alcohol dehydrogenase activity and first pass metabolism. *New England Journal of Medicine, 322*, 95–99.

Galbicka, G., Lee, D. M., & Branch, M. N. (1980). Schedule-dependent tolerance to behavioral effects of delta-9-THC when reinforcement frequencies are matched. *Pharmacology, Biochemistry and Behavior, 12*, 85–91.

Gentry, R., Baraona, E., & Lieber, C. (1990). *Chronic alcohol consumption accelerates gastric emptying and increases peak blood ethanol in rats.* Abstract No. 151, Fifth Congress of the International Society for Biomedical Research on Alcoholism, Toronto.

Goldberg, L. (1943). Quantitative studies of alcohol tolerance in man. The influence of ethyl alcohol on sensory, motor and psychological functions referred to blood alcohol in normal and habituated individuals. *Acta Physiologica Scandinavica, 5*(Suppl. 16), 1–128.

Goldberg, L., & Havard J. (1968). *Research on the effects of alcohol and drugs on driver behaviour and their importance as a cause of road accidents.* Paris: Organization for Economic Cooperation and Development.

Goldman, M., Brown, S., & Christiansen, B. (1987). Expectancy theory: Thinking about drinking. In H. Blane & K. Leonard (Eds.), *Psychological theories of drinking and alcoholism* (pp. 181–226). New York: Guilford.

Goldstein, D. (1972). Relationship of alcohol dose to intensity of withdrawal signs in mice. *Journal of Pharmacology and Experimental Therapeutics, 180*, 203–215.

Goldstein, D. (1976). Pharmacological aspects of physical dependence on ethanol. *Life Sciences, 18*, 553–562.

Goodwin, D. W. (1971). Two species of alcoholic blackout. *American Journal of Psychiatry, 127*, 1665–1670.

Goodwin, D. W., Othmer, E., Halikas, J. A., & Freemon, F. (1970). Loss of short term memory as a predictor of the alcoholic "blackout." *Nature, 227*, 201–202.

Goodwin, D. W., Powell, B., Bremer, D., Hoine, H., & Stern, J. (1969). Alcohol and recall: State-dependent effects in man. *Science, 163,* 1358–1360.

Goodwin, D. W., Schulsinger, F., Hermansen, L., Guze, S.B., & Winokur, G. (1973). Alcohol problems in adoptees raised apart from alcoholic biological parents. *Archives of General Psychiatry, 28,* 238–243.

Goudie, A. J., & Emmett-Oglesby, M. W. (1989). Tolerance and sensitization: Overview. In A.J. Goudie & M.W. Emmett-Oglesby (Eds.), *Psychoactive drugs: Tolerance and sensitization* (pp. 1–13). Clifton, NJ: Humana Press.

Gould, D., Weinberg, R., & Jackson, A. (1980). Mental preparation strategies, cognitions, and strength of performance. *Journal of Sport Psychology, 2,* 329–339.

Greizerstein, H. B., & Smith, C. M. (1973). Development and loss of tolerance to ethanol in goldfish. *Journal of Pharmacology and Experimental Therapeutics, 187,* 391–399.

Grilly, D. (1989). *Drugs and human behavior.* Boston: Allyn & Bacon.

Hagen, R. E., Williams, R. L., & McConnell, E. L. (1979). The traffic safety impact of alcohol abuse treatment as an alternative to mandating license controls. *Accident Analysis and Prevention, 11,* 275–291.

Hall, J. F. (1982). *An invitation to learning and memory.* Boston: Allyn & Bacon.

Harger, R. N., & Forney, R. B. (1963). The aliphatic alcohols. In A. Stolman (Ed.), *Progress in chemical toxicology* (Vol. 1, pp. 53–134). New York: Academic Press.

Haubenreisser, T. (1985). *Acute tolerance to alcohol: Influence of behaviourial variables.* Unpublished PhD thesis, University of Waterloo, Waterloo, Ontario.

Haubenreisser, T., & Vogel-Sprott, M. (1987). Reinforcement reduces behavioral impairment under an acute dose of alcohol. *Pharmacology, Biochemistry and Behavior, 26,* 29–33.

Hawkins, R. D., Kalant, H., & Khanna, J. M. (1966). Effects of chronic intake of ethanol on rate of ethanol metabolism. *Canadian Journal of Physiology and Pharmacology, 44,* 241–257.

Heifetz, S. A., & McMillan, D. E. (1971). Development of behavioral tolerance to morphine and methadone using the schedule-controlled behaviour of the pigeon. *Psychopharmacologia, 19,* 40–52.

Hinson, R. E., & Poulos, C. (1981). Sensitization to the behavioral effects of cocaine: Modification by Pavlovian conditioning. *Pharmacology, Biochemistry and Behavior, 15,* 559–562.

Hinson, R. E., Poulos, C., & Cappell, H. (1982). Effects of pentobarbital and cocaine in rats expecting pentobarbital. *Pharmacology, Biochemistry and Behavior, 16,* 661–666.

Hinson, R. E., & Siegel, S. (1980). Contribution of Pavlovian conditioning to ethanol tolerance and dependency. In H. Rigter & J. C. Crabbe (Eds.), *Alcohol tolerance and dependence* (pp. 181–199). Amsterdam: Elsevier/ North Holland Biomedical Press.

Hinson, R. E., & Siegel, S. (1986). Pavlovian inhibitory conditioning and tolerance to pentobarbital-induced hypothermia in rats. *Journal of Experimental Psychology, 12*, 363–370.

Hoffman, P., Ritzmann, R., Walter, R., & Tabakoff, B. (1978). Arginine vasopression maintains ethanol tolerance. *Nature, 276*, 614–616.

Holden, C. (1991). Probing the complex genetics of alcoholism. *Science, 251*, 163–164.

Hull, J., & Bond, C. (1986). Social and behavioral consequences of alcohol consumption and expectancy: A meta-analysis. *Psychological Bulletin, 99*, 347–360.

Hurst, P. M., & Bagley, S. K. (1972). Acute adaptation to the effects of alcohol. *Quarterly Journal of Studies on Alcohol, 33*, 358–378.

Isbell, H., Fraser, H. F., Wikler, A., Belleville, R. E., & Eisenmann, A. (1955). An experimental study of "rum fits" and delirium tremens. *Quarterly Journal of Studies on Alcohol, 16*, 1–33.

Jaffe, J. H. (1970). Drug addiction and drug abuse. In L. S. Goodman & A. Gilman (Eds.), *Pharmacological basis of therapeutics* (4th ed., pp. 276–313). Toronto: Macmillan.

Jellinek, E. M. (1960). *The disease concept of alcoholism.* New Brunswick, NJ: Hillhouse Press.

Jones, B. M., & Vega, A. (1972). Cognitive performance measured on the ascending and descending limb on the blood alcohol curve. *Psychopharmacologia, 23*, 99–114.

Jones, I. S., & Lund, A. K. (1986). Detection of alcohol-impaired drivers using a passive alcohol sensor. *Journal of Police and Science Administration, 14*, 153–160.

Julien, R. M. (1981). *Primer of drug action* (3rd ed.). San Francisco: W.H. Freeman.

Kalant, H. (1971). Absorption, diffusion, distribution, and elimination of ethanol: Effects on biological membranes. In B. Kissin & H. Begleiter (Eds.), *The biology of alcoholism* (Vol. 1, pp. 1–62). New York: Plenum.

Kalant, H. (1975). Biological models of alcohol tolerance and physical dependence. In M. M. Gross (Ed.), *Alcohol intoxication and withdrawal* (pp. 3–13). New York: Plenum.

Kalant, H. (1987). Tolerance and its significance for drug and alcohol dependence. In L. S. Harris (Ed.), *Problems of drug dependence* (National Institute on Drug Abuse Research Monograph No. 76, pp. 9–19). Washington, DC: U.S. Government Printing Office.

Kalant, H., & Khanna, J. M. (1980). Environmental–neurochemical interactions in ethanol tolerance. In M. Sandler (Ed.), *Psychopharmacology of alcohol* (pp. 107–120). New York: Raven Press.

Kalant, H., LeBlanc, A. E., & Gibbins, R. J. (1971). Tolerance to, and dependence on, some non-opiate psychotropic drugs. *Pharmacological Reviews, 23*, 135–191.

Kamin, L. J. (1969). Predictability, surprise, attention, and conditioning. In B. A. Campbell & R. M. Church (Eds.), *Punishment and aversive behavior* (pp. 279–298). New York: Appleton-Century-Crofts.

Katz, J. L., & Goldberg, S. R. (1987). Second-order schedules of drug injection. In M. A. Bozarth (Ed.), *Methods of assessing the reinforcing properties of abused drugs* (pp. 105–116). New York: Springer-Verlag.

Khanna, J. M., Kalant, H., Sharma, H., & Chau, A. (1990). *Initial sensitivity, acute tolerance and alcohol consumption in Fischer 344 and Long Evans rats.* Abstract No. 318, Fifth Congress of the International Society for Biomedical Research on Alcoholism, Toronto.

Kimble, G. A. (1950). Evidence for the role of motivation in determining the amount of reminiscence in pursuit rotor learning. *Journal of Experimental Psychology, 40,* 248–253.

Kirsch, I. (1985). Response expectancy as a determinant of experience and behavior. *American Psychologist, 40,* 1189–1202.

Kivlahan, D. R., Marlatt, G. A., Fromme, K., Coppel, D. B., & Williams, E. (1990). Secondary prevention with college drinkers: Evaluation of an alcohol skills training program. *Journal of Consulting and Clinical Psychology, 58,* 805–810.

Knight, L. J., Barbaree, H. E., & Boland, F. J. (1986). Alcohol and the balanced-placebo design: The role of experimenter demands in expectancy. *Journal of Abnormal Psychology, 95,* 335–340.

Kopun, M., & Propping, P. (1977). The kinetics of ethanol absorption and elimination in twins and supplementary repetitive experiments in singleton subjects. *European Journal of Clinical Pharmacology, 11,* 337–344.

Krank, M. (1989). Environmental signals for ethanol enhance free-choice ethanol consumption. *Behavioral Neuroscience, 103,* 365–372.

Krasnegor, N. A. (1978). Introduction. In N. A. Krasnegor (Ed.), *Behavioral tolerance: Research and treatment implications* (National Institute on Drug Abuse Research Monograph No. 18, pp. 1–3). Washington DC: U.S. Government Printing Office.

Langenbucher, J. W., & Nathan, P. E. (1983). Psychology, public policy, and the evidence for alcohol intoxication. *American Psychologist, 38,* 1070–1077.

Le, A .D., Kalant, H., & Khanna, J. M. (1986). Influence of ambient temperature on the development and maintenance of tolerance to ethanol-induced hypothermia. *Pharmacology, Biochemistry and Behavior, 25,* 667–672.

Le, A. D., Kalant, H., & Khanna, J. M. (1989). Roles of intoxicated practice in the development of ethanol tolerance. *Psychopharmacology, 99,* 366–370.

Le, A. D., Khanna, J. M., & Kalant, H. (1984). Effect of treatment dose and test system on the development of ethanol tolerance and physical dependence. *Alcohol, 1,* 447–451.

Le, A. D., Khanna, J. M., Kalant, H., & LeBlanc, A. E. (1981). The effects of lesions in the dorsal, median and magnus raphe nuclei on the development of tolerance to ethanol. *Journal of Pharmacology and Experimental Therapeutics, 218,* 525–529.

Le, A. D., Poulos, C. X., & Cappell, H. (1979). Conditioned tolerance to the hypothermic effect of ethyl alcohol. *Science, 206,* 1109–1110.

LeBlanc, A. E., Gibbins, R. J., & Kalant, H. (1973). Behavioral augmentation of tolerance to ethanol in the rat. *Psychopharmacologia, 30,* 117–122.

LeBlanc, A. E., Gibbins, R. J., & Kalant, H. (1975a). Acute tolerance to ethanol in the rat. *Psychopharmacologia, 41,* 43–46.

LeBlanc, A. E., Gibbins, R. J., & Kalant, H. (1975b). Generalization of behaviorally-augmented tolerance to ethanol, and its relation to physical dependence. *Psychopharmacologia, 44,* 241–246.

LeBlanc, A. E., Kalant, H., & Gibbins, R. J. (1976). Acquisition and loss of behaviorally augmented tolerance to ethanol in the rat. *Psychopharmacology, 48,* 153–158.

Leigh, B. (1987). Evaluations of alcohol expectancies: Do they add to prediction of drinking patterns? *Psychology of Addictive Behaviors, 1,* 135–139.

Leino, V. A. (1990). Alcohol use and aging: An evaluation of drinking patterns and life changes. *Drinking and Drug Practices Surveyor, 23,* 25. (Abstract, 14th Annual Alcohol Epidemiology Symposium)

Li, T.-K. (1983). The absorption, distribution, and metabolism of ethanol and its effects on nutrition and hepatic functions. In B. Tabakoff, P. Sutker, & C. Randall (Eds.), *Medical and social aspects of alcohol abuse* (pp. 47–77). New York: Plenum.

Lovinger, D., White, G., & Weight, F. (1989). Ethanol inhibits NMDA-acitvated ion currents in hippocampal neurons. *Science, 243,* 1712–1724.

MacAndrew, C., & Edgerton, R. (1969). *Drunken comportment: A social explanation.* Chicago: Aldine.

Mackenzie-Taylor, D., & Rech, R. H. (1991). Cellular and learned tolerances for ethanol hypothermia. *Pharmacology, Biochemistry and Behavior, 38,* 29–36.

Maisto, S. A., Connors, G. J., & Sach, P. R. (1981). Expectation as a mediator in alcohol intoxication: A reference level model. *Cognitive Therapy and Research, 5,* 1–18.

Mann, R. E. (1980). *Studies of behavioural tolerance to alcohol in male social drinkers.* Unpublished PhD thesis, University of Waterloo, Waterloo, Ontario.

Mann, R. E., & Vogel-Sprott, M. (1981). Control of alcohol tolerance by reinforcement in nonalcoholics. *Psychopharmacology, 75,* 315–320.

Mansfield, J. G., & Cunningham, C. (1980). Conditioning and extinction of tolerance to the hypothermic effect of ethanol in rats. *Journal of Comparative and Physiological Psychology, 94,* 962–969.

Mansfield, J. G., Benedict, R. S., & Woods, S. C. (1983). Response specificity of behaviorally augmented tolerance to ethanol supports a learning interpretation. *Psychopharmacology, 79,* 94–98

Marlatt, G. A., & Gordon, J. R. (Eds.). (1985). *Relapse prevention: Maintenance strategies in the treatment of addictive behaviors.* New York: Guilford.

Marlatt, G. A., & Rohsenow, D. (1980). Cognitive processes in alcohol use: Expectancy and the balanced placebo design. In N. K. Mello (Ed.), *Advances in substance abuse* (pp. 159–199). Greenwich, CT: JAI Press.

Mayfield, D. G., & Montgomery, D. (1972). Alcoholism, alcohol intoxication, and suicide attempts. *Archives of General Psychiatry, 27*, 349–353.

Maynert, E. W., & Klingman, G. I. (1960). Acute tolerance to intravenous anaesthetics in dogs. *Journal of Experimental Therapeutics, 128*, 192–200.

McKim, W. (1991). *Drugs and behavior* (2nd ed.). Englewood Cliffs, NJ: Prentice Hall.

McMillan, D. E., Harris, L. S., Frankenheim, J. M., & Kennedy, J. S. (1970). 1-Δ⁹-*trans*-tetrahydrocannabinol in pigeons: Tolerance to the behavioral effects. *Science, 169*, 501–503.

Meichenbaum, D. (1977). *Cognitive-behavior modification*. New York: Plenum.

Mellanby, E. (1919). *Alcohol: Its absorption into and disappearance from the blood under different conditions* (Special Report Series Monograph No. 31). London: Medical Research Committee.

Mello, N. K., & Mendelson, J. H. (1965). Operant analysis of drinking patterns of chronic alcoholics. *Nature, 206*, 43–46.

Mello, N. K., & Mendelson, J. H. (1970). Experimentally induced intoxication in alcoholics: A comparison between programed and spontaneous drinking. *Journal of Pharmacology and Experimental Therapeutics, 173*, 101–116.

Mendelson, J. H., & Mello, N. K. (1966). Experimental analysis of drinking behavior of chronic alcoholics. *Annals of the New York Academy of Science, 133*, 828–845.

Mendelson, J. H., Stein, H., & Mello, N. (1965). Effects of experimentally induced intoxication on metabolism of ethanol-1-C14 in alcoholic subjects. *Metabolism, 14*, 1255–1266.

Miller, N. E., & Carmona, A. (1967). Modification of a visceral response, salivation in thirsty dogs, by instrumental training with water reward. *Journal of Comparative and Physiological Psychology, 63*, 1–6.

Nathan, P. E., Lowenstein, L. M., Solomon, P., & Rossi, A. M. (1970). Behavioral analysis of chronic alcoholism: Interaction of alcohol and human contact. *Archives of General Psychiatry, 22*, 419–430.

Nathan, P. E., & O'Brien, J. S. (1971). An experimental analysis of the behavior of alcoholics and nonalcoholics during prolonged experimental drinking: A necessary precursor of behavior therapy? *Behavior Therapy, 2*, 455–476.

Nathan, P. E., O'Brien, J. S., & Lowenstein, L. M. (1971). Operant Studies of chronic alcoholism: Interaction of alcohol and alcoholics. In W. McIsaac & P. Creaven (Eds.), *Biological aspects of alcohol* (pp. 341–370). Austin: University of Texas Press.

Nathan, P. E., Titler, N. A., Lowenstein, L. M., Solomon, P., & Rossi, A. M. (1970). Behavioral analysis of chronic alcoholism. *Archives of General Psychiatry, 22*, 419–430.

National Safety Council. (1968). *Alcohol and the impaired driver*. Chicago: American Medical Association.

Newlin, D. B. (1986). Conditioned compensatory response to alcohol placebo in humans. *Psychopharmacology, 88*, 247–251.

Newlin, D. B., & Thomson, J. B. (1990). Alcohol challenge with sons of alcoholics: A critical review and analysis. *Psychological Bulletin, 103*, 383–402.

Newman, H., & Card, J. (1937a). The nature of tolerance to ethyl alcohol. *Journal of Mental Disorders, 86*, 428–440.

Newman, H., & Card, J. (1937b). Duration of aquired tolerance to ethyl alcohol. *Journal of Pharmacology, 59*, 249–252.

Newton, C. (1978). *Motor-skill performance under alcohol as a function of age and drinking experience.* Unpublished MASc thesis, University of Waterloo, Waterloo, Ontario.

Nutrition Canada. (1973). *Nutrition: A national survey* (Project NIP 745–0651). Ottawa: Information Canada.

Ogurzsoff, S., & Vogel-Sprott, M. (1976). Low blood alcohol discrimination and self-titration skills of social drinkers with widely varied drinking habits. *Canadian Journal of Behavioural Science, 8*, 232–242.

Overton, D. A. (1972). State-dependent learning produced by alcohol and its relevance to alcoholism. In B. Kissin & H. Begleiter (Eds.), *The biology of alcoholism: Vol 2. Physiology and behavior* (pp. 193–217). New York: Plenum.

Overton, D. A. (1984). State dependent learning and drug discriminations. In L. L. Iverson, S. D. Iverson, & S. H. Snyder (Eds.), *Handbook of psychopharmacology* (Vol. 18, pp. 59–127). New York: Plenum.

Oxendine, J. (1969). Effect of mental and physical practice on the learning of three motor skills. *Research Quarterly, 40*, 755–763.

Peele, S. (1989). *Diseasing of America: Addiction treatment out of control.* Toronto: Lexington Books.

Pernanen, K. (1976). Alcohol and crimes of violence. In B. Kissin & H. Begleiter (Eds.), *The biology of alcoholism: Vol. 4. Social aspects of alcoholism* (pp. 351–444). New York: Plenum.

Poulos, C. X., & Hinson, R. (1982). Pavlovian conditional tolerance to haloperidol catalepsy: Evidence of dynamic adaptation in the dopaminergic system. *Science, 218*, 491–492.

Poulos, C. X., Hinson, R., & Siegel, S. (1981). The role of Pavlovian processes in drug tolerance and dependence: Implications for treatment. *Addictive Behaviors, 6*, 205–211.

Poulos, C. X., Wilkinson, D. A., & Cappell, H. (1981). Homeostatic regulation and Pavlovian conditioning in tolerance to amphetamine-induced anorexia. *Journal of Comparative and Physiological Psychology, 95*, 735–746.

Preusser, D. F., Ulmer, R. G., & Adams, J. R. (1976). Driver record evaluation of a drinking driver rehabilitation program. *Journal of Saftey Research, 8*, 98–105.

Rangel, J. (1985, July 20). Defendant in mass slaying is guilty of reduced charge. *New York Times*, p. 9.

Rawana, E. (1984). *The influence of reinforcement on the transfer of alcohol tolerance in male social drinkers.* Unpublished PhD thesis, University of Waterloo, Waterloo, Ontario.

Rawana, E., & Vogel-Sprott, M. (1985). The transfer of alcohol tolerance, and its relation to reinforcement. *Drug and Alcohol Dependence, 16,* 75–83.

Rawlings, E. J., Rawlings, J. I., Chen, S. S., & Yilk, M. D. (1972). The facilitating effects of mental rehearsal in the acquisition of rotor pursuit tracking. *Psychonomic Science, 26,* 71–73.

Rescorla, R. A. (1967). Pavlovian conditioning and its proper control procedures. *Psychological Review, 74,* 71–80.

Rescorla, R. A. (1987). A Pavlovian analysis of goal-directed behavior. *American Psychologist, 42,* 119–129.

Rescorla, R. A. (1990a). Instrumental responses become associated with reinforcers that differ in one feature. *Animal Learning and Behavior, 18,* 206–211.

Rescorla, R. A. (1990b). The role of information about the response–outcome relation in instrumental discrimination learning. *Journal of Experimental Psychology: Animal Behavior Processes, 16,* 262–270.

Rescorla, R. A., & Colwill, R. M. (1989). Associations with anticipated and obtained outcomes in instrumental learning. *Animal Learning and Behavior, 17,* 291–303.

Rescorla, R. A., & Wagner, A. R. (1972). A theory of Pavlovian conditioning: Variations in the effectiveness of reinforcement and non-reinforcement. In A. H. Black & W. F. Prokasy (Eds.), *Classical conditioning* (pp. 64–99). New York: Appleton-Century-Crofts.

Richardson, A. (1967a). Mental practice: A review and discussion. Part I. *Research Quarterly, 38,* 59–107.

Richardson, A. (1967b). Mental practice: A review and discussion. Part II. *Research Quarterly, 38,* 265–273.

Ritchie, J. (1985). The aliphatic alcohols. In A. G. Gilman, L. S. Goodman, T. W. Rall, & F. Marad (Eds.), *The pharmacological basis of therapeutics* (pp. 372–386). New York: Macmillan.

Rohsenow, D. J., & Marlatt, G. A. (1981). The balanced placebo design: Methodological considerations. *Addictive Behaviors, 6,* 107–122.

Rush, B. (1814). *An inquiry into the effects of ardent spirits upon the human body and mind with an account of the means of preventing and the remedies for curing them.* Brookfield: Merriam Press.

Salzberg, P.M., & Klingberg, C. L. (1983). The effectiveness of deferred prosecution for driving while intoxicated. *Journal of Studies on Alcohol, 44,* 299–306.

Schmidt, R. A. (1988). *Motor control and learning: A behavioral emphasis* (2nd ed.). Champaign, IL: Human Kinetics.

Schuckit, M., Goodwin, D. W., & Winokur, G. (1972a). The half-sibling approach in a genetic study of alcoholism. In M. Roff & M. Pollack (Eds.), *Life history research in psychopathology* (Vol. 2, pp. 120–127). Minneapolis: University of Minnesota Press.

Schuckit, M., Goodwin, D. W., & Winokur, G. (1972b). A study of alcoholism in half-siblings. *American Journal of Psychiatry, 128,* 1132–1136.

Schuster, C. R., Dockens, W., & Woods, J. (1966). Behavioral variables affecting the development of amphetamine tolerance. *Psychopharmacologia, 9,* 170–182.

Schwartz, B. (1978). *Psychology of learning and behavior.* New York: W. W. Norton.

Schwartz, B., & Lacey, H. (1982). *Behaviorism, science and human nature.* New York: W. W. Norton.

Sdao-Jarvie, K. (1988). *The role of response expectancies in the acquisition and display of alcohol tolerance.* Unpublished PhD thesis, University of Waterloo, Waterloo, Ontario.

Sdao-Jarvie, K., & Vogel-Sprott, M. (1986). Mental rehearsal of a task before or after ethanol: Tolerance facilitating effects. *Drug and Alcohol Dependence, 18,* 23–30.

Sdao-Jarvie, K., & Vogel-Sprott, M. (1991). Response expectancies affect the acquisition and display of behavioral tolerance to alcohol. *Alcohol, 78,* 491–498.

Sdao-Jarvie, K., & Vogel-Sprott, M. (in press). Learning alcohol tolerance by mental or physical practice. *Journal of Studies on Alcohol.*

Seitz, H., Egerer, G., & Simanowski, U. (1990). Letter to the Editor. *New England Journal of Medicine, 323,* 58.

Shapiro, A., & Nathan, P. (1986). Human tolerance to alcohol: The role of Pavlovian conditioning processes. *Psychopharmacology, 88,* 90–95.

Sher, K. J. (1985). Subjective effects of alcohol: The influence of setting and individual differences in alcohol expectancies. *Journal of Studies on Alcohol, 46,* 137–146.

Shortt, R. G., & Vogel-Sprott, M. (1978). Social drinkers' self-regulation of alcohol intake. *Journal of Studies on Alcohol, 39,* 1290–1293.

Shortt, R. G., & Vogel-Sprott, M. (1981). Monitoring blood alcohol concentrations: Hypotheses and implications for alcoholism. *Journal of Studies on Alcohol, 42,* 350–354.

Siegel, S. (1975). Evidence from rats that morphine tolerance is a learned response. *Journal of Comparative and Physiological Psychology, 89,* 498–506.

Siegel, S. (1976). Morphine analgesic tolerance: Its situation specificity supports a Pavlovian conditioning model. *Science, 193,* 323–325.

Siegel, S. (1977). Morphine tolerance acquisition as an associative process. *Journal of Experimental Psychology: Animal Behavior Processes, 3,* 1–13.

Siegel, S. (1978). A Pavlovian conditioning analysis of morphine tolerance. In N. A. Krasnegor (Ed.), *Behavioral tolerance: Research and treatment implications* (National Institute on Drug Abuse Research Monograph No. 18, pp. 9–19). Washington, DC: U.S. Government Printing Office.

Siegel, S. (1979). The role of conditioning in drug tolerance and addiction. In J. D. Keehn (Ed.), *Psychopathology in animals: Research and treatment implications* (pp. 143–168). New York: Academic Press.

Siegel, S. (1989). Pharmacological conditioning and drug effects. In A. J. Goudie & M. W. Emmett-Oglesby (Eds.), *Psychoactive drugs* (pp. 115–169). Clifton, NJ: Humana Press.

Siegel, S., Hinson, R. E., & Krank, M. D. (1978). The role of predrug signals in morphine analgesic tolerance: Support for a Pavlovian conditioning model of tolerance. *Journal of Experimental Psychology: Animal Behavior Processes, 4,* 188–196.

Siegel, S., & Sdao-Jarvie, K. (1986). Attenuation of ethanol tolerance by a novel stimulus. *Psychopharmacology, 88,* 258–261.

Simpson, H. (1975). *Analysis of fatal traffic crashes in Canada, 1973. Focus: The impaired driver.* Ottawa: Traffic Injury Research Foundation.

Smode, A. F. (1958). Learning and performance in a tracking task under two levels of achievement information feedback. *Journal of Experimental Psychology, 56,* 297–304.

Sobell, M. B., Sobell, L. C., & VanderSpek, R. (1979). Relationships among clinical judgement, self-report, and breath-analysis measures of intoxication in alcoholics.*Journal of Consulting and Clinical Psychology, 47,* 204–206.

Speisky, M. B., & Kalant, H. (1985). Site of interaction of serotonin and desglycinamide-arginine-vasopressin in maintenance of ethanol tolerance. *Brain Research, 326,* 281–290.

Staiger, P., & White, J. (1988). Conditioned alcohol-like and alcohol-opposite responses in humans. *Psychopharmacology, 95,* 87–91.

Stewart, J., DeWit, H., & Eikelboom, R. (1984). The role of unconditioned and conditioned drug effects in the self-administration of opiates and stimulants. *Psychological Review, 91,* 251–268.

Suzdak, P. D., Glowa, J. R., Crawley, J. N., Schwartz, R. D., Skolnick, P., & Paul, S. M. (1986). A selective imidazobenzodiazepine antagonist of ethanol in the rat. *Science, 234,* 1243–1248.

Suzdak, P. D., Glowa, J. R., Crawley, J. N., Skolnick, P., & Paul, S. M. (1988). Is ethanol antagonist Ro15-4513 selective for ethanol? *Science, 239,* 649–650.

Tabakoff, B., & Hoffman, P. L. (1988). Tolerance and etiology of alcoholism: Hypothesis and mechanism. *Alcoholism: Clinical and Experimental Research, 12,* 184–186.

Tabakoff, B., Ritzman, R. F., Raju, T. S., & Deitrich, R. A. (1980). Characterization of acute and chronic tolerance in mice selected for inherent differences in sensitivity to ethanol. *Alcoholism, Clinical and Experimental Research, 4,* 70–73.

Thompson, R. F., & Voss, J. F. (Eds.) (1972). *Topics in learning and performance.* New York: Academic Press.

Thurman, R. G., Cheren, I., Forman, D., Ewing, J. A., & Glassman, E. (1989). Swift increase in alcohol metabolism in humans. *Alcoholism: Clinical and Experimental Research, 13,* 572–576.

Tolman, E. C. (1932). *Purposive behavior of animals and men.* New York: Appleton-Century-Crofts.

Truitt, E. B. (1971). Blood acetaldehyde levels after alcohol consumption by alcoholic and nonalcoholic subjects. In W. McIsaac & P. Creaven (Eds.), *Biological aspects of alcohol* (pp. 212–232). Austin: University of Texas Press.

Vaillant, G. E. (1983). *The natural history of alcoholism.* Cambridge, MA: Harvard University Press.

Vestal, R. E., McGuire, E. A., Tobin, J. D., Andres, R., Norris, A. H., & Mezey, E. (1977). Aging and ethanol metabolism. *Clinical and Pharmacological Therapeutics, 21,* 343–354.

Vingilis, E., Adlaf, W., & Chung, L. (1982). Comparison of age and sex characteristics of police-suspected imparied drivers and roadside-surveyed impaired drivers. *Accident Analysis and Prevention, 14,* 425–430.

Vogel-Sprott, M. (1975). Self-evaluation of performance and ability to discriminate blood alcohol concentrations. *Journal of Studies on Alcohol, 36,* 1–10.

Vogel-Sprott, M. (1979). Acute recovery and tolerance to low doses of alcohol: Differences in cognitive and motor skill performance. *Psychopharmacology, 61,* 287–291.

Vogel-Sprott, M. (1983). Response measures of social drinking: Research implications and applications. *Journal of Studies on Alcohol, 44,* 817–836.

Vogel-Sprott, M. (1986). *Behavioral tolerance to alcohol: Expectancies and incentives.* Paper presented at the meeting of the American Psychological Association, Washington, DC

Vogel-Sprott, M., & Barrett, P. (1984). Age, drinking habits and the effects of alcohol. *Journal of Studies on Alcohol, 45,* 517–521.

Vogel-Sprott, M., & Fillmore, M. (1991). *The placebo response to alcohol: A three expectancy problem?* Unpublished manuscript, University of Waterloo, Waterloo, Ontario.

Vogel-Sprott, M., Kartechner, W., & McConnell, D. (1989). Consequences of behaviour influence the effect of alcohol. *Journal of Substance Abuse, 1,* 369–379.

Vogel-Sprott, M., Rawana, E., & Webster, R. (1984). Mental rehearsal of a task under ethanol facilitates tolerance. *Pharmacology, Biochemistry and Behavior, 21,* 329–331.

Vogel-Sprott, M., & Sdao-Jarvie, K. (1989). Learning alcohol tolerance: The contribution of response expectancies. *Psychopharmacology, 98,* 289–296.

Vogel-Sprott, M., Sdao-Jarvie, K., & Fillmore, M. (1991). *Response expectancies affect acute tolerance and the profile of impairment under alcohol.* Unpublished manuscript, University of Waterloo, Waterloo, Ontario.

Vuchinich, R. E., & Tucker, J. A. (1983). Behavioral theories of choice as a framework for studying drinking behavior. *Journal of Abnormal Psychology, 92,* 408–416.

Vuchinich, R. E., & Tucker, J. A. (1988). Contributions from behavioral theories of choice to an analysis of alcohol abuse. *Journal of Abnormal Psychology, 97,* 181–195.

Vuchinich, R. E., Tucker, J. A., & Rudd, E. J. (1987). Preference for alcohol consumption as a function of amount and delay of alternative reward. *Journal of Abnormal Psychology, 96,* 259–263.

Wagner, A. R., & Rescorla, R. A. (1972). Inhibition in Pavlovian conditioning: Application of a theory. In R. A. Boakes & M. S. Halliday (Eds.), *Inhibition and learning* (pp. 310–337). New York: Academic Press.

Wallgren, H., & Barry, H. III. (1971). *Actions of alcohol*. Amsterdam: Elsevier.

*Webster's new collegiate dictionary*. (1973). Springfield, MA: Merriam-Webster.

Wenger, J. R., Berlin, V., & Woods, S. C. (1980). Learned tolerance to the behaviorally disruptive effects of ethanol. *Behavioral and Neural Biology, 28*, 418–430.

Wenger, J. R., Tiffany, T. M., Bombardier, C., Nicholls, K., & Woods, S. C. (1981). Ethanol tolerance in the rat is learned. *Science, 213*, 575–577.

Wilson, J., & Crowe, L. (in press). Genetics of alcoholism: Can youth at risk be identified? And should we? *Alcohol Health and Research World*.

Wise, R. A. (1988). The neurobiology of craving: Implications for the understanding and treatment of addition. *Journal of Abnormal Psychology, 97*, 118–132.

Wise, R. A., & Bozarth, M. A. (1987). A psychomotor stimulant theory of addiction. *Psychological Review, 94*, 469–492.

Wolgin, D. L. (1989). The role of instrumental learning in behavioral tolerance to drugs. In A. J. Goudie & M. W. Emmett-Oglesby (Eds.), *Psychoactive drugs: Tolerance and sensitization* (pp. 17–114). Clifton, NJ: Humana.

Wolverton, W. R., & Schuster, C. R. (1978). Behavioral tolerance to cocaine. In N. A. Krasnegor (Ed.), *Behavioral tolerence: Research and treatment implications* (National Institute on Drug Abuse Research Monograph No. 18, pp. 127–141). Washington, DC: U.S. Government Printing Office.

Worden, J. K., Flynn, B. S., Merrill, D. G., Waller, J. A., & Haugh, L. D. (1989). Preventing alcohol-impaired driving through community self-regulation training. *American Journal of Public Health, 79*, 287–290.

Worobec, T. G., Turner, W. T., O'Farrell, T. J., Cutter, H. S., Bayog, R. D., & Tsuang, M. T. (1990). Alcohol use by alcoholics with and without a history of parental alcoholism. *Alcoholism: Clinical and Experimental Research, 14*, 887–892.

York, J. (1990). Letter to the Editor. *New England Journal of Medicine, 323*, 59–60.

Zinatelli, M. (1992). *Drug-free learning enhances alcohol tolerance in humans*. Unpublished PhD thesis, University of Waterloo, Waterloo, Ontario.

Zinatelli, M., & Vogel-Sprott, M. (1990). Learned tolerance to alcohol: Mental rehearsal with imagined consequences. *Alcoholism: Clinical and Experimental Research, 14*, 518–521.

Zusman, M. E., & Huber, J. D. (1979). Multiple measures and the validity of response in research on drinking drivers. *Journal of Safety Research, 11*, 132–137.

# Index

217